WOUNDED HEALER

FRONTIERS IN PSYCHOTHERAPY SERIES
Edward Tick, *Series Editor*

Freud & Cézanne: Psychotherapy as Modern Art, *by Alexander Jasnow*

Gestalt Voices, *edited by Edward W.L. Smith*

Gestalting Addiction: The Addiction-Focused Group Therapy of Dr. Richard Louis Miller, *by Angela Browne-Miller*

Hope Under Siege: State Terror vs. Family Support in Chile, *by Michele Ritterman*

The Many Colored Buffalo, *by William S. Taegel*

Transcending Addiction and Other Afflictions: Lifehealing, *by Angela Browne-Miller*

Walking Wounded—Men's Lives During and Since the Vietnam War, *by Steve Trimm*

Wounded Healer, *by John Gagnon*

in preparation

My Father was Shiva, *by James Flosdorf*

Relational Psychotherapy in Practice, *by Robert Willis*

WOUNDED HEALER

by

John Gagnon

ABLEX PUBLISHING CORPORATION
Norwood, New Jersey

Printed in the United States of America

Library of Congress Cataloging-in-Publication Data

Gagnon, John.
Wounded healer / by John Gagnon.
p. cm. -- (Frontiers in psychotherapy series)
ISBN 0-89391-973-X (cl). -- ISBN 1-56750-063-3 (ppk)
1. Psychotherapists--Mental health--Case studies. 2. Gagnon, John. 3. Amputees--United States--Biography. 4. Testis--Cancer--Patients--United States--Biography. I. Title. II. Series.
RC451.4.P79G34 1993
616.89'0092--dc20
[B] 93-44570
CIP

Ablex Publishing Corporation
355 Chestnut Street
Norwood, New Jersey 07648

I dedicate this book lovingly to Carolyn and Isabelle.

CONTENTS

ACKNOWLEDGMENTS

I wish to acknowledge many wonderful healers, physicians, nurses, therapists, dear friends and clients: The off duty EMTs on Route 7 in June of 1981, the ambulance crews from Ridgefield and Danbury, Craig Foster, Robert Cooper, Robert Reiffel, the staff nurses at the Danbury and White Plains hospitals, Jay Weiner, those who donated blood on my behalf, Ron Raymond, George Anderheggen, Ralph Welsh, George Steinfeld, Fran and Alan Stave, Bob and Nancy Weston, Ed and Karen Santella, Janet Swift, Ed Schewe, Ted Peatte, Ernie, Fay, Susan, and Ken Gagnon, Pauline Gagnon, Ray, Elex, Ray Jr. and Marph Ingersoll, Mario Howell, Asho and Lyle Craine, Michael Clementy, Paul Colella, Virginia Dziedulonis, Sophie Lombardo, Paul, Rose, and Rose Paula Dziedulonis, Tom and Aline Mahon, Florina Mattson, Maryann, Rich, Richy, Jillann, and Cynthia Salkowski, Helen Botti, Ursula Dambrowski, Ann Thorpe, Peggy Daines, Bob and Lois Walsh, George Rogers, Laura Perls, Frank Reissman, June and Bird Volckhausen, Bill, Andrea, Billy, Mike, and Stacey Perillo, Mike and Barbara Searing, Janie Starbuck, Lynn Bernstein, the Bengtsons, Henry Bright, Joanne Davidson, Jonathan Fox and Jo Salas, Vince and Alice Furfaro, Bruce Mardiney, all of Playback Theater, Sam and Nancy Deibler, Paul Doniger, Keith, Marie, Jonathan, and Sara Dupree, Brian Geen, Carolyn Holt, Sharon Joyce, Seabury and Eleanor Lyon, Seabury Lyon Jr. and David Lyon, Susan Mathews, Bill McWilliams, Marcia Geller, John Mickelson, Pam and Stuart Bell, Jan Bidwell, Doug and Ellie Miller, Ed Tick and Kim Roffman, Bruno Stroili, Toby and Merri Gould, Doug

Griffin, Donna Lawrence, John and Elaine Metz, Larry Anderson, Jean and Jerry Renjilian, Dominique and Noel Regney, Allen Mendler, Stan Kline, Bruce Buzby and Gerri Boggs, Wayne and Rosemary Raulerson, Mary Jo, Becky, and Josh Lent, Judy Swallow, Sarah and Will Wechsler, Paul Selgin, Dorothy Towey, Pat Lipovsky, Rita Lisko, John Orlando, Arnie and Diane Pfeil, Jamie and Terry Pfeifer, other friends and acquaintances who visited me in my hospitalizations, the rest of my family at the Unitarian Universalist Society of Northern Fairfield County, Carolyn and Tom Hanes, Owen McManus, Joe Fitzgerald, Michael and Audrey Price Whalen, Kin Carmody, Sarah Partly Cloudy, Gene Eliasoph, Paul Morton, Seb Mucilli, Tom Nissley, Tommy and Susan Aldridge, Judy Yurmark, Pat Dick, Howard Rovics and Anne Chamberlaine, Steve Ross, Vinny Keane, Roberta Wood, Pat Warfield, Rich Borofsky, Darius Brubeck, Jim Whiteside, Sky and Kathy Cole and the gang around Rainbow Lake, Tom Pratt, Bonnie Zielke, Joan North, Kert Southerland, Diana Buckley, my brother and sister learners at the Union Institute, teachers and mentors in emergency care and psychotherapy, the men and women of the Connecticut Emergency Service Association, Billy Demby and the other amputees of the '52 Association, the many EMTs whose lives I have been allowed to touch because of my experiences, the dedicated men and women who are involved in all aspects of emergency services every day of their lives (local, State and Federal) and last, but certainly not least, the literally hundreds of clients who have given my life a sense of continuing purpose in the dark moments and have been a source of personal joy and even inspiration for me as they strived to grow through their own struggles, pain, and suffering.

FOREWORD

The original outline and planning for the book *Wounded Healer* began in the summer of 1987. It was suggested to me by my friend and colleague, Dr. Ralph Welsh. He had told me on a number of occasions that the story of my life over the prior six years would make interesting reading for others. He was especially interested in the way that my writing might be of some use to other psychotherapists who had suffered from traumatic personal losses. While he never suggested directly that the writing of the manuscript might, itself, serve a therapeutic purpose, I suspect that Ralph knew all along that it might be helpful to me to examine the events that had occurred and the ways in which I had responded to them in an effort to integrate emotionally these experiences into my daily living.

I first began by making an outline. This was very useful in getting me into the process of writing the first chapter (I think beginning writing has always been hard for me). The opening story about the accident was relatively easy to do because I wrote the story from the third person. I told *about* myself from the position of observer rather than writing from the locus of a person experiencing an accident. As I wrote, I sometimes felt like I was an EMT at the scene, and I found the emotional distance from the experience useful. It relieved me from having any painful attachments to the memories. The second chapter, however, which actually tells the story from my own perspective, was quite different.

I often found myself stopping in order to cry, sometimes softly, sometimes wailingly. The pain was great and was not yet finished. As each revision of the personal chapters was completed, I found the emotional attachment and mourning decreased. There was a true relief. Remembering the smaller details turned out to be a necessary step in my completion of the total grief process for the losses I had suffered. While the reality of pain was met and dealt with in the earlier stages of writing, the meaning to the suffering was not addressed until the beginning of the editing process in 1990. Dr. Ed Tick, editor of *Voices*, offered me a publishing contract with Ablex. I had written about a dozen chapters to my book but had no idea how I was going to end it or what meaning it held.

Ed made some initial suggestions about directions I might take, but a great deal of thanks goes to Kim Roffman, who encouraged me to look at the kinds of alterations that emerged in my personality as a result of being a wounded healer.

At first I had more questions than I had answers. It was not until I had listened to the views and suggestions of my clients, colleagues, and others and reviewed the changes that I could recognize in myself that I came in touch with an even deeper sense of loss and, at the same time, saw the marvelous emotional and spiritual supports that had been there for me. I also realized some things about my unrealistic attitudes in the past. As far as my behavior was concerned, I had a self-view that was almost devoid of vulnerability. I had the erroneous belief that living life as a healer protected me from harm. I had believed, based upon my Catholic upbringing, that if I helped others, nothing bad or painful could ever happen to me. In a way, this created a kind of arrogance in the face of harm. I don't believe that I was a particularly reckless individual, but I do believe that I was blinded by a trust in my own infallibility. The way I dealt with the tractor-trailer taught me that I had to take better care of myself, that the world was not my overly protective parent who would keep me from harm. I also learned that being a "good" person had nothing to do with protection from harm, and that vicissitudes happen to everyone, regardless of the life they lead. I know that I already thought this on an intellectual level, but it took the accident and the cancer to teach this to me on the emotional and psychological levels. There was also a spiritual growth that resulted from my seeing God as the supportive aspect of life rather than as the one who made bad or good things happen to others. Another spiritual component occurred when I could let go of needing to control so much of my life and give in to life's own ebb and flow.

There were times during the writing of the manuscript when I wished that I had achieved some great discovery from my suffering, one that would revolutionize psychotherapy. I think that this was just another way in which I was taking myself for granted and was wanting to substitute a childhood need for acceptance through achievement in place of self-acceptance. By the time I had finished writing, however, I realized that it would be enough to tell the story of the ways in which I had been a human being, a person who had suffered and found ways to heal others, sometimes *because* I had experienced pain. I also learned that I needed to do the work of helping others in order to find meaning in my life after each of my tragedies. My work, therefore, became an extremely important support to me and to my feelings of self-worth. I think that an area of further growth for me has been to see my worth outside of my role as a healer and to experience more pleasure in my life on a simpler basis. Perhaps that journey will be the material for a second book? I'm uncertain. I don't picture myself much as a writer. That you *are* reading this book at all is more due to the encouragement of my friends, colleagues, and editors who have had the patience and interest to proofread the various stages of the manuscript and to make helpful suggestions.

I have learned from them to keep my mind more focused on a particular audience and to deliver my story in a language consistent with that audience. I have learned a great deal about the organizing of years of experience into salient mini-stories which would, in their nature, represent the many other, similar stories that I could have recounted.

I have also learned that the process of writing, like the process of living, is really what is important, more important than any particular outcome, even the completing of a book.

CHAPTER 1

The headline story began with an account of the Ridgefield police officer who had been assigned to the afternoon shift on June 11th, 1981. He had received the dispatcher's message about an accident that had occurred on Route 7 near the Foundry Restaurant. Using his lights and siren, he had driven in his black-and-white cruiser the five miles from his post—in the downtown area near the police station—to the scene within a matter of minutes.

At a location on the road approximately 30 feet north of the tiny stone bridge above Bennett's Farm Road and across from the restaurant sat an eighteen-wheel tractor trailer. It had come to rest slightly in the oncoming lane of traffic and partially on the embankment to the left side of the road. Behind it was a 90-foot diagonal skid mark, suggesting that the truck, laden with crushed car bodies, had been traveling approximately 60 miles per hour on a road marked for a 45-mile-per-hour speed limit. Beneath the second set of double right rear cab tires was the flattened body of the yellow Honda moped on which the accident victim had been riding. The point of impact had been roughly opposite to the entrance of Bennett's Farm Road in the oncoming traffic lane of the state road. The tank and wheels of the moped had been crushed. They were almost perfectly flat due to the massive weight of the truck.

Immediately following the collision, traffic began to back up both in the north- and southbound lanes of the road. Several people came out of the Foundry Restaurant. Others ran from two tiny gift stores and Al's

Coffee Shop, a small diner situated above the restaurant, when they heard the crash. Two of these persons put in calls for police and the ambulances. Fortunately for the moped rider, however, there were also, stuck in the lines of traffic, several off-duty EMTs. When they learned what had taken place ahead of them, they grabbed their jump-kits (the boxes in which first-aid equipment is stored) and came to the aid of the rider.

They reported finding the rider seated upright in a wide puddle of blood in the road, holding onto the stump of his severed left leg. He was apparently in shock as he did not respond to them when they spoke to him and soon passed out when one of them touched him.

While Danbury and Ridgefield EMS were en route, these off-duty EMTs applied pressure to arteries of the left leg and to the crushed right leg as well. The truck-cab front tires had evidently passed over both legs, and the rear tires caught and trapped both moped and rider beneath them, carrying him for a distance of approximately 30 feet. The results on the rider of the abrasion of the tires and the macadam road, as well as the crushing effect of the weight of the truck, were an almost spontaneous amputation of the left leg, the breaking of all of the ankle, foot and toe bones of the right foot, a crushing or communuted fracture of the tibia and fibula of the right leg, a dextroversion of the right foot (turning it around so that it pointed backwards), and the removal of all skin and some of the muscle and lymph tissue from the ankle and right foot. When they cut the rider's wallet out of the brown, vinyl jacket they found his name on the driver's license: John Gagnon.

When the medical technicians identified me, I was totally unconscious with a blood pressure of about 70 over 50 and in an advanced state of hypovolemic shock (a condition due to the loss of blood). They say that the unconscious mind can still record the things that people say, and I did recall later some words spoken by one of the EMTs while I was in this unfortunate state.

When the Ridgefield ambulance arrived, the medics from this service, who were all IVs—trained in the intravenous administration of fluids—took not only the large, orange first-aid boxes called "trauma kits" from their ambulance, but also a two-foot-long "D" tank of oxygen and several plastic bags of clear saline solution.

By this time the puddle of blood in the road was larger. I had lost several units of the precious, life-sustaining liquid. My breathing was very rapid but scarcely visible, and the IVs later reported that my chest barely rose and fell. One fellow thought I might have stopped breathing altogether.

In spite of the drama of the scene, the approaching EMT–IVs had to thoroughly assess things. They opened up the already cut areas of clothing with their large, shear-like scissors and saw the tangled left leg. Intravenous needles with hollow, plastic lines were immediately inserted into the rapidly collapsing veins of the right arm, and the precious saline solution began to do its job of keeping those veins open for the blood I would receive when I got to the hospital emergency room. They said later that they knew that this was a "haul and carry" situation, another name for a circumstance so serious as to require immediate transport with lights and siren. With blood leaving the body, there were fewer and fewer red cells to carry oxygen to the brain and other tissues. In a short time the whole toxic, irreversible process of severe hypovolemic shock would set in, and I would simply have died of oxygen starvation. To help with the lowered oxygen-carrying capacity of the blood, they also inserted a special airway into my throat. The tube carried the forced oxygen deep into the lungs where, with each shallow breath, I would get as much of the vital, life-sustaining gas as possible.

While the oxygen was set up, I was later told that another of the off-duty medics pulled a hand full of 4″ × 4″ gauze pads from his kit. He said that he made certain to keep the pads sterile, took a pair of long tweezers and a bottle of saline solution and proceeded to the crushed moped. There he began the grisly task of picking up the bone fragments that lay about in the road. Washing the blood and street dirt off each piece with the saline, he placed the splinter in a gauze pad and set it in a pile. When he had picked up all of the larger pieces, he lifted the gauze and returned to the ambulance where he placed the small bone bundle in an emesis basin for the trip to the emergency room.

Despite the urgency everyone reported feeling about me, the IVs from Ridgefield, Joe and Ken, knew that more bleeding could start if they didn't get a fast assessment of the other injuries. The secondary examination was brief. The right foot was turned around backwards and had no flesh or lymph tissue left on it. This is also known as a "degloving injury," a softer description of the nasty avulsion of skin and muscle that made the foot look like a shank of pork in a store window.

Apparently, when one of the onlookers saw the foot, she was so overcome by the sight that she passed out and had to be treated by one of the Danbury EMTs who had arrived next. Right after this, a news reporter and photographer from a Danbury paper arrived and began writing and taking pictures of what would be tomorrow's feature story.

The ambulance personnel also noticed that the right leg was twisted and shortened, a sign that either the thigh bone or the two lower leg bones were broken and compacted. The former injury would be a bit more serious since a broken femur can cut the main artery to the leg and the rest of the body's blood can leak into the muscles of the upper leg, finishing off the process of bleeding to death. A look at the exposed thigh assured the ambulance crew chief that the fractures were all confined to the lower leg, to the tibia and fibula. That completed the secondary survey and prepared me for transport to the hospital.

One of the off-duty EMTs plus two more from the Danbury ambulance pulled out the stretcher. They had tugged the release lever and lowered the pallet to the ground, ready to receive my limp body. One last look at the head and spine showed that the back and neck were not broken, but there was already a bleeding and swelling contusion on my forehead that might tell of further brain damage.

They carefully lifted me onto the stretcher and then raised it so it could be wheeled over to the back doors of the Ridgefield ambulance. On the stretcher I was held in place with nylon belts with velcro fasteners. I later learned that at the moment they lifted me up I woke again. Apparently it is not unusual for persons in shock to act quite agitated, and I began to move my arms around. Even though they were partly restrained by the straps, I was able to flail them upward. This risked dislodging the precious IV line. Ken grabbed my hands and pinned them down. Joe, Michael, Dave, and Allen lifted the stretcher up, locked it into place in the special holding bracket in the ambulance, and the Ridgefield team jumped in for the ride to Danbury Hospital.

Once in the ambulance, Joe attempted to see if I was responsive. This would aid in maintaining a level of consciousness in the event that I did have brain damage or was slipping into deeper shock. Again I moved. This time my whole body went into motion. I violently leaned upward, straining against the nylon straps. My face contorted in a mindless grimace. I whimpered and growled (inasmuch as this was allowed by the airway in my throat) meaningless animal sounds. My strength seemed incredible to the two attending EMTs. Ken immediately leaned over me and rested his entire weight diagonally on my chest as the ambulance steadily wove its way closer to the emergency room. Joe communicated with the hospital by radio throughout the rest of the trip, giving them the vital information they needed to receive their new patient. The emergency room would be prepared for a "shock-trauma victim with crushing injuries to both legs."

Someone had to inform my wife, Carolyn, and my daughter, Isabelle, that I had been in an accident. Ted Peatte, a friend of mine with whom I had met earlier that same fateful day, decided he would do it. He arrived at the small, brown, wooden cottage on the edge of Rainbow Lake in Ridgefield a little after 4 p.m. When he first knocked on the door, no one responded and he was almost going to leave when my daughter finally answered. Isabelle was 9 years old at that time and was a little wary of Ted even though she had seen him on a few previous occasions.

Ted struggled with the difficult task of convincing Isabelle to fetch her mother without telling the child directly that anything horrible had happened to me. Finally my daughter told him that Carolyn had gone to bed so she could get some sleep before she went on night shift at the hospital (where she was a nurse in the neonatal unit), and that she did not want to be disturbed "under any circumstances." Apparently, Isabelle persisted at some length in obeying her mother's instructions but Ted eventually managed to convince her that the news he had was very important. My daughter told me later that she really didn't want to wake her mother, but she finally did it because Ted "wouldn't go away." Ted remembers that he was quite concerned about how to say things and wondered what it would be like for his wife to hear what he was about to say to Carolyn.

Moments later, Carolyn Gagnon stumbled into the light. She obviously had been asleep by the look of her eyes and her tousled hair. When she asked what the visit was about, Ted told her that I had been in an accident while on the moped. Carolyn asked what had happened to me and Ted had some difficulty finding a way to put it. He finally told her that I had been hit by a tractor-trailer, but that I was going to live. He told her that the truck had run over the lower part of my body and that the EMTs to which he had spoken had some doubts whether the doctors at Danbury Hospital could save my legs.

Carolyn then wanted to know if Ted had been with me or had seen the accident. He told her that we had met earlier but that we had agreed to get together back at my house later so Ted could take me down to see his wife's new store on Mamanasco Lake. Ted, who was an EMT and fire fighter, said that he had heard of the accident because he was listening to his police-fire scanner when the call came in. He then drove up Route 7 to see if he could assist with anything, got around the traffic jam by using his emergency light, and was thoroughly shocked to see that the victim was me.

When Carolyn asked him if I was in the hospital, she appeared "kind of spacey." It was as if she had become psychologically numbed to the news, and I imagine that this was her own natural defense against dealing with the entirety of the tragedy all at once. Ted then offered to drive her to the hospital and, though Carolyn agreed to this offer of help, she first wished to place Isabelle with neighbors and to leave a message on the answering machine for anyone who called before she got back home.

The Lents were not only neighbors but had become very close family friends to all of us. Becky and Isabelle were playmates and Carolyn and MaryJo were very good friends. Carolyn decided to call them. Wesley, MaryJo's husband, answered the phone but was very quick to deal with Carolyn's concerns about Isabelle and agreed to keep Isabelle for an indefinite period of time until Carolyn was emotionally ready to be with her again. Carolyn found this to be quite a relief and was then able to turn her attention to getting dressed and preparing herself dispassionately to see me in the hospital. The last thing that my wife did was to record a very detailed message on the answering machine. In it she told the caller that I had been in an accident and that the person could call the Lents for further information. She knew that her parents were out of town, visiting their son in New Mexico and that if they called they would want to know what had happened. Carolyn later described her efficiency as "being on automatic pilot." After setting the machine to receive calls, she left with Ted.

As Ted turned the car onto Ridgebury Road, away from Route 7, Carolyn asked him why he chose to go to the hospital by a rather obscure back route. He replied that he did not want her to see the blood in the road. She remembers feeling grateful for his sensitivity.

When I arrived at the hospital, the stretcher was quite soaked in blood. The IV team had succeeded in keeping my veins open and in keeping the bleeding down to a minimum, but I had still lost a considerable volume. They carried bags of saline solution above the level of the stretcher in their hands as I was wheeled down to the E.R. bays. I didn't know it at the time, but the only parking spaces available next to the ambulance parking area were handicapped spaces. I would become very familiar with these spaces from this day forward.

A nurse met the stretcher inside the entrance way and pointed toward the double doors leading to the treatment bays. The gurney was wheeled rapidly around corners, down the light green hallway and into the room that had been prepared for bone injuries. Part of the reason for this haste is something called "The Golden Hour." This chronological unit is the time limit that a medical team has in which to save the life of a trauma victim who is in severe shock.

With ER interns giving orders the nurses began the task of cleaning out the wounds. One green-cloaked ER nurse depressed the plunger on an antiseptic solution, washing the exposed muscles. One of the EMTs later described "a stream of sandy, clot-choked, reddish liquid that ran onto the ER floor." A phlebotomy technician took a sample of blood and ran it down to Blood Bank where it was quickly typed and cross-matched. Bags of B+ packed blood cells were rushed back to the emergency room and prepared for the operating room. I would need thirteen units before the surgery was completed that night. Within minutes after a call from one of the interns, a young, tall, fair-haired orthopedic surgeon rushed into the room. Dr. Craig Foster was on call the afternoon of June 11th, 1981 to handle any orthopedic or traumatic injuries brought into the ER. After a brief examination of my injuries, he quickly ordered that the operating room be prepared for surgery. He immediately requested other capable surgeons in the fields of microsurgical technique, neurology, and anesthesia.

Carolyn was not allowed into the emergency treatment area at first. Instead, she was led into Dr. George Terranova's office. The head of the ER sat on his desk as he told her that I was going to live but that I had been quite seriously injured and had lost a great deal of blood. Everything he said only increased her numbness, but she found this protective. He then informed her that I would probably have to lose at least one and possibly both of my legs in the surgery that would soon take place. Carolyn remembers that although she was intellectually cognizant of what he said, she was too emotionally anesthetized to respond to him during his progress report.

After a while Dr. Foster came into Terranova's office. There was some blood on his white lab coat, she noticed. Then she saw that he was a tall and young-looking man. She had mixed feelings at first but his voice "...his voice was so...soothing, so comforting," she later told me. She relaxed a little as he told her that the operating room had been prepared and that I would have to suffer an amputation of the left leg. He also presented her with a number of forms and permission sheets which she, being the spouse, would have to sign for the surgery.

Carolyn immediately refused to sign anything that had to do with amputation. She was willing to give permission for exploratory or reconstructive surgery but amputation was another thing.

Foster explained that it was commonplace for the spouse to assume responsibility for such operative procedures following a severe traumatic injury or whenever the patient was unable to assume responsibility for himself, but she stubbornly persisted.

She emphasized again that exploratory or reconstructive surgery was "acceptable," but amputation was not. She knew that they had attempted to get the various bits and pieces of the appendage from the road and she wanted him to try to reassemble my left leg if at all possible. Also, she did not know Craig Foster, nor of his reputation as a surgeon, and she did not want him doing the wrong thing. She planned to call around for the best surgeons in the area as soon as she got back to MaryJo's.

Seeming to understand at least part of her concerns, he told her that for this procedure, at any rate, they would not do an amputation and would try to save both legs. He then asked her if she wanted to visit with me. He told her that I was stable and could see her for a few moments. She followed Foster into the trauma room. I was lying on the stretcher. Carolyn remembers seeing the vague form of a man she once recognized. There was a large contusion on the forehead under my brown hair and the sheets tucked around me were spotted red in contrast to the grey-green color of my body. The scene took on a nightmare quality for her. It was real, but at the same time not real. I was picking up my head in an attempt to look at my feet and then collapsing back onto the pillow. I am told that I spoke to no one, though several people had tried to get some kind of response from me. Carolyn swam forward through a sea of concern to the side of the pallet. I was looking around but not seeing. Her words to me were kind and soft.

I don't remember them, but she told me much later that she said, "John, I'm here with you. I love you very much." She also touched my arm, below the IV tube. This apparently had some sort of calming effect on me. I seemed to relax a bit. I then sank onto the stretcher, let go and slipped back into sweet, painless unconsciousness.

Next, Ted Peatte came into the room and also tried to speak to me. I neither heard Ted nor moved. He was about to turn away when something on the floor caught his eye. Bending down, he picked up a white stick and showed it to Dr. Foster. Foster said something and Ted lay the leg bone on the stretcher next to my side. He stepped back, blinking the tears from his eyes. The transport team then gathered around the table and lifted my body onto the gurney headed for operating room number four.

A nurse in "preop," sterile in her green gown, inserted a syringe into my arm at the elbow. Despite the efforts of the IV team to inflate the blood vessels, it was difficult to find the vein. Finally, the needle in place, she inserted the new IV line. In my particular case, there was no need for pre-anesthetic. I was already at so much risk by being in shock that I didn't need to have my central nervous system depressed any further. The heart and lungs might stop altogether. They had to get more blood into me immediately, however. She hung the bags of bright red liquid on the poles stuck in the side of the table.

The anesthesiologist, also dressed in the usual green scrubs of the OR, placed a black rubber mask over my pale face. As the EKG technician hooked up his equipment to monitor the already weakened heart, the scrub nurse set out the necessary instruments for the operation. Foster prepared for the work, his mind already in surgery. He told me later that he didn't think he could save the left leg but that he was certainly going to do everything that was medically possible. There simply wasn't much tissue left to work with.

Five hours later, the orthopedic surgeon, his green shirt and pants soaked with sweat, his back aching with the strain of leaning over the operating table, stepped back to allow the "assisting" to close up the last repair on the left leg. Three separate surgical teams had been working simultaneously. They had done all that they could do for that limb. Foster moved over to the lower left side of the table and, picking up his camera, took the last flash picture of the uncovered leg in its metal frame. The entire procedure was recorded for future medical reference.

Blood was steadily oozing out of the contorted flesh. It would be dressed later. He then went around to the other side of the operating table and carefully unwrapped the gauze from the denuded and twisted right ankle. As soon as he saw the foot he realized that it was easily as much of a problem as the severed leg. There was so much crushing that important blood vessels might have been damaged and might make amputation on this side necessary as well. When I think of the many hours of work he had done on the left leg I can only imagine the weary frustration that the right ankle presented to him. But he persevered.

The foot had to be rotated back to the forward-facing position and microsurgically reconnected to a few significant veins and arteries. The removal of skin and connective tissue would not be addressed in this operation. Once the blood flow was established, the foot was temporarily rewrapped and enclosed in a partial cast to prevent any damage from movement. Another entire piece of surgery would have to be done to finish the job. That would wait until I was physically stronger.

The left leg then looked like something that a child might mold out of clay to resemble that piece of human anatomy. It was slightly amorphous and was shrouded in blood-soaked bandages. It was held together by a frame of steel rods and pins. By a little after midnight, Foster was cleaned up and ready to follow my semiconscious form up to ICU.

The intensive care unit (ICU) can be a nerve-wracking place for a new employee to work. There are so many sights and sounds, all related to life-and-death situations. Special EKG machines called "cardiac monitors" give regular auditory signals and visual graphs corresponding to the contractions of various chambers of the heart. Numbers representing pulse rate and blood pressure (from indwelling transducers) are on display. Byrd respirators aid some patients to breathe, their regular "clack…puff…clack…puff" becoming a normal, background part of the din of life-supporting noise. There are humming, rattling auto-infusion pumps which pass very accurately measured quantities of medications, saline, glucose, blood cells, or hyper-alimentation (liquid nutrients) into the bodies of some patients. On a rare occasion there is the shrill scream of an alarm in the cardiac monitor. This occurs when the heart of the patient being monitored stops for some reason. When a patient's heart stops, ICU personnel and others in the area of the "code" (as this emergency situation is called) come running to start CPR, "push" bicarb, get cardiac stimulants going and intubate and "bag" the comatose, arrested patient. They will try to reverse the dying process and restore him/her to the company of the living once again. Many ICUs have a high burnout and turnover rate.

At half-past midnight, Carolyn met Foster in the ICU. He was there with three nurses who were trying to make me as comfortable as possible under the circumstances. My body was angled to one side. The gauze bandage on the leg was already soaked through, but they would not try to change it that night. They would, instead, keep hanging the bags of packed B+ cells and bags of whole blood containing clotting agents. The first thing that Carolyn noticed was that the entire room smelled of blood.

Foster commented on my condition: stable. Carolyn then told him what she had done. Being a nurse she recognized the need for a quick response to this emergency, and she wanted to be absolutely certain that I would receive the best medical care available. When she had returned to the Lent's she immediately started to call friends and relatives to get the names of important trauma surgeons in the New York area.

Doctors from Yale, Albert Einstein, The Hospital for Special Surgery, and other equally reputable places were named to Carolyn. She reached many of them by telephone. Several people mentioned capable physicians from Columbia Presbyterian. At the same time, other members of Carolyn's family started giving advice about an attorney for a law suit, but she persisted in getting information about physicians. Cornell's staff of elite surgeons were added to her list. She had not yet reached any decisions.

Carolyn did not recount to Foster that she had also attempted to call an old family friend who was professor of orthopedic surgery at Columbia, Charlie Neer. Charlie was not in at the time. He would know who to recommend. She'd have to try again tomorrow.

Foster concluded their conversation by informing her that they had done just about all they could do in that operation and that he would call a friend of his at Bellevue who was the chief resident of microsurgery. Apparently, Foster wanted to examine additional ways to increase patency in the left leg and to get his opinion about further surgery on the right foot. Throughout this "visit" I kept moaning as the nurses continued to straighten out the linen on my bed.

Carolyn was startled when Foster's pager went off. He automatically reached down to his belt, unclipped the offending noise-maker and walked to the phone by the bed. The operator told him that he was wanted in ER, something about "a crushed hand." That would be another couple of hours for him. As he turned to leave, I stirred. Without thrashing, without so much distance in my eyes, I wrestled to get my head up off of the pillow. I had no idea what was happening at this time. Staring straight ahead I spoke through a hoarse and parched throat my first words since the accident.

"What am I doing here? What's happened?" I said quite coherently, although I am told that I seemed to be in a great deal of pain.

Before anyone else in the room could speak or even move to keep the woman from approaching the bed, Carolyn slipped past the nurse to her right and stepped up to the edge of the lowered left bed rail. Placing both of her hands firmly on my shoulders she spoke to me. Her words this time, unlike the time in the ER examination area, were not kind or soft. They were direct and honest but, apparently, the effect was the same. I relaxed once again and slipped back onto the pillow. I let out a long sigh and closed my eyes. I remained motionless, and my breathing became regular.

At 2 a.m., Craig Foster got a phone call from Bellevue. He stepped out of the OR, unscrubbed and went to a desk phone. A lengthy conversation ensued in which Foster discussed every piece of my surviving anatomy with his friend. The colleague asked dozens of questions about the health of various tissues, especially in the circulatory system. When Foster hung up he knew that he had done everything he could have for me. He also knew what course of action he would be taking next. He redressed, scrubbed and went back into surgery to work on the tendons in the new patient's crushed hand.

It was almost midmorning before Foster awoke in the on-call room provided for overnight staff at the hospital. He told me later that his back reminded him of the night he'd had. He washed up, failed to shave, changed his clothes and headed for the cafeteria for a cup of coffee. Unlike most mornings, when a cup of "hospital mud" usually woke him up, he was still tired when he left.

He eased the B.M.W. into the driveway and tiptoed up the front steps as if he might disturb someone. He knew that everyone would be up by then—it was already 11:30 a.m.—but it was a habit. His wife Kathy was in the kitchen. She was used to Craig getting home at strange hours when he was on call. Usually it was 2 or 3 a.m.

Craig didn't speak. He walked to the bathroom without a word, hesitated, turned toward Kathy, jerked forward, she says, and "burst into tears." He spoke about the young man on whom he had operated last night. He was very concerned about me. When I think about this, I am always deeply moved by his show of human emotions.

Carolyn met with Connie, the Clinical Director of Surgery at the hospital. She told Connie about the list of surgeons she had acquired. She also told her that she wanted the best person for me even if that meant moving me someplace else. She wished that Charlie Neer would return her calls because he had such a good reputation and knew so many fine orthopedic surgeons.

When Carolyn mentioned Charlie's name, Connie seemed extremely surprised. She told Carolyn that she had scrubbed for him when she worked in the operating room at Columbia Presbyterian.

They spent some time discussing what a fine surgeon he was, and Carolyn told her that Charlie had been an old friend of the family. Carolyn then suggested that maybe Charlie could recommend someone in the area who was a better orthopod than Foster. Carolyn said Connie was quite surprised at this and told her, "You've already *got* the best in the area. Foster was Charlie's surgical Fellow!"

The second piece of surgery I underwent was on the right foot. When it was completed, the area from several inches above the ankle down to the mid-foot was still denuded of flesh, but it was well supported in a steel Hoffman Apparatus, a kind of cage that allowed all of the eighteen broken bones to stay in place around the various screws, inserted rods, and plates that would act as temporary support until the bones knitted together once again. The five dislocated and broken bones had been straightened, many arteries and veins had been reconnected by the microsurgeon, and there was a slight increase in blood-flow to and from the foot. It was nothing short of a medical miracle.

Completing a routine check of vital signs, the nurse turned back toward me. Carolyn watched her glance fall first to the foot of the bed. Both legs were in traction. Carolyn's attention was drawn by the blood-soaked bandages on the left leg. She knew that my leg was quite a mess and she felt her first pangs of doubt that they would be able to save it.

"Hello," said the nurse.

"Hello," I am told I responded almost a bit too brightly.

Carolyn stood back, waiting for the nurse to finish her mental status examination, checking to see how oriented I was to person, place, and time.

"Do you know your name?" The nurse poised her pen above the form clipped to my chart.

"Yep," I replied in a curt manner.

"All right then," she said, sounding as if she was irritated with me. "What is your name?"

"John!" I smiled now despite what was an incredible amount of pain. They had been giving me regular injections of morphine throughout the night in response to my moans.

"Very well, John. Can you tell me where you are now?"

"Yep," I replied in the same, simple, assured manner.

"Yes…well then…where are you?"

"In California!" I apparently said in the same firm, simple and yet totally confident way.

Carolyn stepped forward and said softly to the nurse, “I guess he needs to be in California right now.”

I'm glad that I have no personal recollection of this incident, but it does seem a bit amusing in retrospect.

CHAPTER 2

"What a positively gorgeous day this is," I thought to myself as I looked through the wide windows that completely surrounded the office attached to the garage. The bright blue sky was filled with story-book clouds. I knew that as soon as I finished with my last client for the day that I would just have to take the moped out for a ride. This was one of those perfect days that only happens a few times during the year, and I wanted to take advantage of it.

The first three sessions went rather well. I was feeling good and it showed in my therapy. I seemed to be one step ahead of each of the clients who had arrived so far, seeing exactly where each one was going to go in the therapeutic moment before he or she got there.

I would get a late lunch today at Ted's place, the Foundry Restaurant just about 2 miles away on the other side of Route 7. I called Ted and arranged to meet him there at 2 o'clock. Albert arrived exactly at noon. He would be my last client for the day.

Albert Milton was a 45-year-old salesman for a major electronics company. He had held many jobs in sales but often got fired for doing something "wrong." Once, when he was selling used cars, Albert promised the same car, taking deposits both times, to two separate customers. They complained to the boss and Albert pleaded that his error was completely unintentional. He had made so many "errors" like this, however, that his boss immediately fired him.

I looked at Albert as he entered the room. As a Gestalt therapist, I always begin my work the moment I first lay eyes on the client for the session. Sometimes I am amazed at how the entire theme for the session is disclosed by the unconscious mind in those first few, unguarded moments.

For example, one woman came into a first session and said in the principal moment of meeting, "I sure hope this isn't going to cost much." For the next seven months of her therapy we were constantly dealing with her unwillingness to make any effort (pay anything) on her part in order to change. She wanted change and growth just to happen. She also expected her relationships to improve without her "paying" anything into the relationship. It took her over ten sessions to finally catch on to the way in which she lived her life (passively) and to realize that she *had to pay* for the things that she wanted. She had given me the metaphor for her work in the open door she provided in the first few seconds of our meeting.

When Albert arrived, he looked flushed, apprehensive, frightened. He glanced around the room as if afraid that someone might be watching him before he took his seat on the green couch opposite the hard folding chair on which I preferred to sit (it always keeps me alert).

"You look quite shook-up today, Bert. What's going on?"

Leaning forward onto his elbows, Albert stared at the oriental carpet. He seemed to be in a trance for a moment as if he was seeing a scene in his mind. Then he slowly raised his head and spoke, "I remembered something yesterday evening. I've been thinking about it most of the night." He paused.

I nodded and urged him to go on.

"Well...I was watching a program on T.V. about some guy who was always...uh...it was a movie...always in some kind of trouble with his boss, wife...you know...everybody. He was a grown up version of 'Peck's Bad Boy.' I realized right then and there that I was just like him...I mean...that's not any kind of news. We've known about my getting into trouble for weeks now...but I remembered something else this time." He stopped again.

"Remembered what, Bert?" I looked at his hands. They were twisting and wringing one another. Finally his hands went under his coat which was folded in his lap.

"I remembered that I was always getting into trouble at school when I was a kid. I mean, that doesn't sound like a 'divine revelation' or anything considering how I can't keep a job these days but...it was like no matter how much I tried to do the rights things, I was always in some kind of trouble. It would seem to just *happen* to me!"

"Would just happen?"

"Yeah. I never wanted to get into trouble. I never thought about it. There were these other kids. They were always getting into trouble but they wanted to. They enjoyed doing trouble-making things to the teachers. Not me, though. I never wanted to cause anyone any problems. I always wanted to be a 'good boy,' the teacher's pet but I never could be. The harder I tried the worse things got."

"Do you understand why you always acted in such a way that you got *yourself* into trouble?" I said this to emphasize his sense of responsibility for his own life.

"No. That's what disturbs me. It's like I was always trying so hard to be good, to do the right thing and it just didn't matter."

Thinking about his hands under the coat and the way he entered the room (trying to hide) I said, "If you could have hidden from someone in your childhood, who would you have liked to get away from?"

He look startled when I said that. I persisted. "I mean, was there anyone who you needed to hide from who was constantly watching you as a child?"

Now Albert began to shake. He looked again at the ground. "My mother," was all he said.

"So you wanted to hide from your mother?"

"Yeah. She was always looking to see what I was doing. She followed me around the house all of the time. I never knew where she would turn up next." His hands relaxed and came out from under the coat. They lay in a comfortably folded position in Albert's lap.

"Your mother *spied* on you a lot. Is that it, Bert?"

"Yes. She was often looking into the doorway of my room and checking up on me."

"As if she didn't trust you?"

"That's it, as if..." Albert paused again and stared at the center of the oriental rug.

"What are you thinking of right now?"

"Oh...um...I was just thinking that she *never* trusted me."

"That thought had just occurred to me as well."

"Yeah, but what does that have to do with what I came in to tell you about today?" Albert genuinely looked perplexed.

Getting an idea, I decided to change this from an intellectual speculation *about* Albert's childhood to an actual experiential reliving of something from his childhood.

"Give me a moment, Bert," I said. I needed to think about how to reproduce in the therapeutic process an experience that would duplicate what his mother might have done to him. I had it.

"Bert, would you be willing to try something for a moment?"

"Depends on what that is."

"Well, you know how I sometimes ask you to relive early life experiences that you had as a child in order to learn more about them? (He nodded). Well, I would like you to go back to your childhood right now and relive something about your mother's spying. O.K.?"

"O.K. I'll try it. What do you want me to do?"

"I would like you to imagine that this room is actually the room you had as a child. If that were the case, then I would like to know where various things were...are...in the room; the bed, the desk—if you had one—other objects. You tell me where they would be."

Albert stood up slowly and wiped his hands on his pants. They didn't look sweaty but he acted as if they were. Then in general terms and as time went on in more specific detail he pointed out where every one of his things would be if this was his room. When he had finished he looked entranced. I had seen that look before. He was actually seeing the room as if it was his old bedroom.

"You see it, don't you?"

"Yeah. It's kind of weird, but for a moment I felt like I was a kid again."

"O.K., Bert. So, if you *are* a kid and this *is* your room and the couch is the bed like you indicated, I'd like you to tell me what you are doing on one occasion when your mother is spying on you."

Albert moved toward the "bed" and sat on the edge of it. He noticed his coat and pushed it off to one side. My guess was that he didn't want that object to distract him from his reverie. His eyes glazed slightly as he tried to remember. After a while he spoke. "I was once sitting on my bed doing something. I don't know what it was. I was playing or something like that."

"Playing? Playing with what?" I was wondering if he had been masturbating. I remembered once being found masturbating by *my* mother and what an embarrassing experience it had been.

"I don't know...something...paper...and I think that I was also on the telephone at the same time."

"So, you had something made of paper...a book maybe?"

"Yeah a book or a...magazine! That's it. I had some kind of magazine."

Following a hunch I went to my "prop closet" and pulled out a copy of Playboy. "Could it have been a copy of a magazine like this one?"

Albert's face got red when he saw it. "I...I think so."

"And who would you be talking on the phone with...right now as you sit on your bed?"

"I think it was one of the other boys."

"So, you might have been sitting on the bed, looking through a magazine and talking to one of your friends. Is that right?"

"Could be. I think so.... Yes."

"Wait a minute." I went back to the prop closet and got out a regular black cradle phone and handed it to him. "Take this and imagine that you are talking to your friend. What might you be saying?"

Albert reached for the phone and rested it beside himself on the "bed." He took the receiver off of the cradle and held it up to his left ear, craning his neck over to the left in order to hold the phone in place. With his left hand he opened the magazine and turned instinctively to the centerfold. When he felt natural in the position he began. "Hello, Bill? Wait 'till you see the babe in this month's Playboy. God, she's fantastic. She's got this skimpy 'baby-doll' top on and no underpants. She's a real knock-out." Immediately Albert began to look embarrassed and frightened.

"What's happening now?"

"My mother is standing in the doorway." Albert got a bit pale as he said this.

"And what is she doing?"

"She is…she's yelling at me. She is calling me all kinds of names…painful names." Albert began to sound a bit choked up and his eyes were getting wet. He sucked in his breath and turned his face away from me.

"You look sad right now, Bert." I felt real compassion in my heart for this "young boy."

Biting his lip, he muttered, "No…not really. Well, maybe I'm a little sad…a little. Mostly I feel…I don't know what to call it?"

Taking a guess I said, "Humiliated? Would you call it humiliated?"

"Yeah!! That's it exactly. I feel real humiliated like I've done something terrible."

"Well, Bert, I would like you to try something else right now. Would you come over here (pointing to the imagined "doorway" of the room) and play your mother for a moment?"

"O.K." Albert got up and, laying down his black cradle phone and magazine, moved to the doorway. He suddenly seemed to grow larger in stature. His face became contorted with anger and his eyes glowed hatefully. Albert began, "You rotten, no good, son-of-a-bitch. You are just like your father. You are a no good pervert! How can you look at that trash. I've heard from my girlfriends about things like this. You are no good. You never were and you never will be!"

"All right, 'mother.' I've got a question for you. Do you see the magazine Bert is reading?"

As mother, Albert looked thoughtfully down at the bare place on my couch which had become the bed in Albert's room so many years ago. "Mother" answered, "No…not exactly…but I know the kind of stuff he would probably read. He's no damn good and never has been!" Albert's face got red and puffy as he spoke. His hands had become fists resting on his hips.

"O.K., Bert. Come back here (to the couch) and answer your mother."

Albert returned, sat down forcefully on the "bed" and immediately burst into tears. "I am not such a bad boy. I'm *not*!! You always say that to me. I am not so bad. I'm really not." Albert then lowered his head and sobbed uncontrollably. I moved over next to him.

"May I touch you, Bert?"

"Yeah," he sobbed and nodded at the same time.

I put my arm around him and he cried even more wrackingly. After a while the muscles of his middle back began to tighten. I sensed a different feeling and pulled away.

"What is happening now, Bert?"

"I feel mad. She's wrong. I don't know why but she's wrong about me."

"Tell this to her." I moved over on the couch at remove from Albert so he could muster his own supports for this confrontation.

Albert raised his head and looked at the far side of the room, his eyes glazed over and he "saw" his mother. "How dare you call *me* 'bad'!! I am *not* bad. You are wrong about me. You were always wrong about me!" Albert was practically screaming here. His hands were grasping at the air as he spoke.

"What do you want in your hands, Bert?"

"I want to hit her with...with the magazine!"

"So pick up the magazine and roll it up or hold it the way you would if you were going to hit her with it. I don't want you to do anything, however."

Albert picked up the magazine and looked at the title. His mouth dropped open, his shoulders hunched forward and he began to sob anew. "This is not the kind of magazine I had that day. It was *Time Magazine* and I was doing my *homework* with my friend, Bill. It wasn't even what she thought!!"

"O.K., Bert. So she found fault with you even when you hadn't done anything wrong."

"Yes...she was *horrible* to me!!" Albert leaned forward and began to cry again. I felt such an empathy for him. Imagine, to be constantly thought of as someone other than who you are. I guess Albert finally began to act out in real life what his mother believed about him all along.

"Bert, do you understand what this might have to do with your frequently doing the 'wrong things' at school and now at work?"

He looked up at me with tear-streaked cheeks and began a natural smile. "Yep. I believe that I must have become the person she saw me as."

"That's right, Bert. That's what I think too. Maybe now you can begin to work on acting in a way that does not fit your mother's image of you. O.K.?"

"That would be nice." He laughed.

Well, I ended the session on this insightful note and after scheduling

Albert for next week I finished up my paperwork for the day.

I looked at my watch. It showed 1:30 p.m. I realized that I could now see Carolyn. We had lived together from 1978 until the present and had fought quite a bit during the first couple of years. We had managed to work out a majority of that stuff. In fact, by June 11th, 1981, we were quite pleased to be with one another. Our problems mostly had to do with how different we were from one another. We had had very little in common and had found this to be a regular source of discontent when we first moved in together. What we had finally discovered was that we complemented one another really well, and what had been a problem with difference became a source of strength for us. We had just gotten married the previous October (1980) and had a great time in New Mexico in December. We were in love. Such a nice place to be after so much arguing. I got up from my desk and went in search of my lovely wife.

"Hello lover," I said as I saw her standing in the bedroom. She looked up at me with her steel-blue eyes and winked. I admired her as she got undressed. I knew she had to go to sleep now so she could get up to work the night shift at the hospital but I was willing to be a little sexually playful anyway. "Come 'ere." I kissed her long and deeply. God, but she turned me on.

"See you later...goodnight," she said. As she sat down on the edge of the bed my thoughts shifted to more responsible notions. I remembered Isabelle. She was Carolyn's daughter from her previous marriage but I had raised her from the age of 6 and she was every bit *my* daughter now. I knew she'd wonder where I was when she got home from school.

"When Isy wakes you up later, tell her that I'll be back around suppertime." Carolyn said she would. I quickly kissed Carolyn, turned and left. I was now eager to enjoy the beautiful weather.

When I got to the garage I reached down and lifted the overhead door. The bright yellow moped was sitting right in the middle of the one-car space. It held a place of honor. Not being one to take large risks I felt like this tiny, 49 cc bike was my "Harley." A one-hour ride on it was the equivalent of a weekend vacation to me. I loved the feeling. I pulled out the choke. Turning on the gas feed I switched the ignition on and began pedaling as fast as I could. The tiny engine started up and the "putt-putt" was the roar of a giant "road machine" to my ears.

I parked it in the driveway only long enough to close the garage door and then hopped on and drove off down Crescent Drive at an exciting rate. The speedometer read 10 mph. I felt the wind in my hair and the warmth of the sun. The lilacs gave the air a sweet and pleasant smell. The geese were at the small, mottled beach at the end of Lakeside Drive. "My goodness," I thought, "how large the goslings have grown!" I was alive and

I felt splendid.

At the bottom of Bennet's Farm Road I stopped the moped. I looked across Route 7 until an opening cleared in the traffic and then moved briskly across the road, entering the driveway to the Foundry. Once inside I looked around for Teddy. Wayne, his brother told me that he wasn't there yet so I ordered up a cheeseburger, medium of course, a plate of fries and a Coke. Wayne and I chatted a bit and, guessing that Teddy had stood me up, I decided to leave. I climbed back on the moped and began driving up the gravel path when Ted appeared. The white Trans Am looked freshly washed and waxed.

"Hey...Where the hell you been?" I said with a laugh.

He spoke through the rolled-down window. "At the lake." He rubbed his hair. "I had to finish up some stuff for Francine. Hey...want to see her new store?"

"Sure. Is this down on Mamanasco?"

"Yeah. You want to follow me?"

"No. Not on this thing. How about I go back to the house and get the car and meet you someplace?"

"How about I meet you at your place and then you can follow from there?"

"Sure. Fine. See you later," I said as he ran the Trans Am down the driveway to turn around. He came by me. I waved and watched him head off into traffic down Route 7. I guessed he had some business to attend to before he met me at the house. I looked out onto the small, two-lane highway. The traffic from the north had subsided and there was only a tractor-trailer coming down the hill to the left.

"O.K.," I thought as I pulled out across Route 7 toward Bennet's Farm Road.

A hazy fog settled over the ship...over the *hull* of the ship as the crews lowered the cargo into my hold...into me. Strong stevedores lifted me up...I was the cargo now..."I've got to hold on...to what?" Something tiny in the black void clawed at my numbed brain. "The hold is full!! I'm shitting...loose, runny shit." Someone wiped my backside. "Oh God!! The pain!!! The hold is full of cattle..." A stampede later, "I am empty now." The haze. The blackness settled in. "There it is again, the thing that claws at me. What does it mean? What is the meaning?" I was a ship in a dark port.

The nurse came swiftly into the room. I was lying on the bed, my left leg or what remained of it supported in its metal frame, the right foot in traction. I was shouting and crying.

"Stop this hurt...the pain!!!! Stop it. Stop it!"

She rubbed the alcohol soaked cotton on the muscle of my right arm and injected the morphine. I stopped yelling after a while and dropped right off into a sleepy delirium again.

I was a church organ. The pipes were tall and hollow. I was making deep, growling music. "Carolyn?...Is that you, Carolyn? It's O.K. I'm fine. I'm studying with this master right now.... I'm learning so much. He's John Henry-like. It's O.K. Don't cry. I am just learning about the mysteries! When I finish studying I'll be home. An accident? Injuries?" I remembered a face coming at me in ICU. It was...it *is* Carolyn's face. She has her hands on my shoulders. "What am I doing here? What happened to me?" I said. She put her hands on my shoulders and said...she said something... something.

The haze parted. "The pain! God, it's so intense!" A white lab coat that hung open like a cape stood in front of me. It was big...tall.

"Hi. I'm Doctor Foster. I'm your surgeon and I've got to ask you for permission for something. O.K.?"

"What's that?" I said rather matter of factly.

"Well, we've done al that we can in trying to save your left leg. Right now the tissue is dying...."

"You mean gangrene?"

"Yes. And the toxic effect will be life-threatening if we don't amputate your leg. Do you understand what I'm saying to you?"

"I do." I rolled the ridiculous dream-like statement over in my fuzzy brain. It was just as absurd as everything else I was experiencing.

The lab coat spoke again. "I asked your wife for permission to amputate, but she wanted you to have the decision. We cut down on your morphine dose so you could be lucid. What do you want us to do?"

"You say that I'll die if I don't have this amputation?"

"Yes. That's a possibility. We're feeding you a lot of antibiotic, but you have such poor circulation that the leg is just dying. We've really got to remove it."

"If you say it has to be done, then do it." I was completely convinced by the logic of it all. The fact that there was a whole emotional component to this decision had not occurred to me at all.

"Are you sure?"

"Yes." A clipboard was placed in front of me. Lots of words on it. So many words. Something about "permission" and "surgery." I signed it before the nurse returned...before the *haze* returned.

"A cast? They put a cast over an amputated stump?" I lay in the bed in the orthopedic ward confused by a plaster cast. I thought they only did things like this for broken bones, not for surgical procedures. I had come to understand that I had had an accident and that I had suffered a serious, crushing injury to my left leg. I also knew that I had nearly lost the right foot as well. "How could this be happening? I don't understand." The face was leaning toward me again. It was...Carolyn's face...I was suddenly back in the ICU. She said something....Finally, I heard the voice as clearly as if she had been standing in the room with me.

"You've had a terrible accident. Your legs are badly injured and you had surgery." I lay back on the pillow and cried like my heart would break. I am crying again as I type this recollection.

The room was clean and neat. There were flowers on the nightstand by the side of the bed. A large metal pole ran the length of the bed and there was a trapeze-like thing hanging from the pole just about two feet above my chest. I guessed I could use that pole to pull myself up in the bed if I needed to. On the opposite wall hung the dozens of cards from friends. Had I read those cards? I didn't remember. Funny how long it took for me to begin to record in memory my being in the hospital. Except for those strange scenes about being a boat and an organ. Oh yes, and being in some kind of training program with a "master" or something. I think I was referring to the male nurse who took care of me during the first few weeks in the orthopedics ward or wherever I was. It was so hard to remember. So many holes. I imagined that the morphine had something to do with it but I wasn't sure. This whole thing seemed so terrible. How could I be riding my moped one second and then the next second be lying in a bed in the hospital with one leg amputated. "Oh yeah...I signed the papers for the surgery." I had remembered something anyway. In fact I more than remembered it. I actually felt grateful to Carolyn for insisting that Foster come to me for the permission. That was a very loving and wise thing for her to do.

When Carolyn visited me she told me that during one bout of delirium after the surgery I had said that I "lost my father, my wife (Sharon, my first wife), and my leg."

Carolyn had thought to herself, "But I'm still alive. I'm here."

She also told me about Craig Foster coming into the room and remarking that he and I were tall guys and my saying, "Not any more! Oh well, I was too tall anyway!" I felt weird hearing my own reactions to the horrible thing that had happened to me. The psychotherapist in my head said, "It is obviously the first stage of the grief process: denial." But I still felt crazy. The whole thing was crazy, wasn't it? How could this have happened to me?

Visitors came and went. I received lots of cards and letters. One of the most impressive came in a large plastic frame. It was a letter from the

American Red Cross describing how many people in Ridgefield and Danbury actually went to a blood mobile and donated blood in my name. This was very touching. Years later, I would meet one of these persons and he would enter therapy with me. In the mean time, whenever I saw a visitor, I was always quite pleasant and charming. This bravado was mostly a sign of denial. When they left I cried. The appearance of pleasantry, however, made me seem much more courageous than I felt.

June 28th was supposed to be the family picnic of 1981. This was a reunion that I organized each year. I used to send out fliers to dozens of family members all over the tri-state area to get them together. We usually took pictures, played games, sang songs, and ate lots of very good, home-cooked, ethnic food (most of the family were either Polish or Italian). It was June 28th. I was told that the families would not be meeting out of deference to my accident. I was irritated. I wanted them to meet anyway. I had gone to all the trouble to organize the picnic again that year. It really meant a lot to me and I wanted my relatives to get together and have a good time. I was disappointed by their decision.

Most days in the hospital were the same. There were the usual visitors, the three forgettable meals, the medications. Come to think of it, I actually used to look forward to those meals, not because of any enjoyable tastes, but because it was another way to pass time. It gave me something to do despite the books, puzzles, games and distractions people brought me. As the denial began to pass I felt myself becoming increasingly more frightened. There was an anger forming in me that was of mammoth proportions. But I just couldn't let it come. I was retroflecting.

Retroflection is the mental act of turning back toward oneself an energy that belongs outward. Some depressions are often the retroflection of anger, and women who have been raised not to express anger are often prone to this type of depression.

Over the past nine years during which I had been a psychotherapist I had witnessed numerous examples of reinforcement for or encouragement of retroflection brought about by institutions established for the mental and physical well-being of patients. Before I became a Gestalt therapist, I was never quite clear about the healthy need for angry and resentful expression, but I often felt uncomfortable with the way in which these feelings were handled in institutional settings. At one mental hospital where I trained, I saw several patients express anger in loud yelling or in punching a piece of furniture. These patients were restrained with camisoles, put in isolation rooms, or tied to their beds. One patient who kicked a standing ash tray over was wrestled down by several aides and put in a strip isolation room in a less "progressive" ward. I remember thinking, "God, if I were in this place I would have lots of reasons to be angry and would want to express this. What are patients supposed to do?" Obviously what they were supposed to do and, in fact, did do was to suppress any expression of angry feelings. Depression was rampant and so were all kinds of psychotic symptoms. I couldn't help but wonder how these patients might have been helped by not only allowing them to express anger but, in fact, even encouraging them to use punching bags, cushions, Batacca bats, or something else to get rid of angry feelings in safe and acceptable ways.

Years later when I directed a program for schizophrenic patients my staff and I found that the Gestalt practice of allowing and facilitating anger and resentment was responsible for reducing depressive and psychotic symptoms in patients we treated. Again, I found that the administrative supervisor in the institution for which I worked (this very hospital) did not support such therapeutic interventions and considered patient behavior "regressive acting out." I was eventually fired for refusal to change my approaches to the successful treatment of these patients.

The more I had learned about the benefits of helping patients to undo the chronic retroflection of angry and resentful feelings the more I facilitated patients in the expression of these feelings. Over the years I often had heard from patients that other treatment settings had discouraged such expressions and always gave them more Thorazine when they showed their honest anger over something.

Throughout my hospitalization I found out that things had not changed at all from those days. I was given Dilaudid for pain, Haldol to calm me down, and Elavil to thwart any depressive symptoms that might develop. I was drugged and foggy most of the time. I found that there was a general acceptance of sadness and crying by nurses but not by my psychiatrist. The psychiatrist sent to "help me out" (on my own request, by the way) would often point out to me that I still "had two arms, was not a spinal cord injury, and was lucky to be alive."

I kept thinking, "I'm not crying for what I've got! I'm crying for what I've lost." I never let anyone at any hospital discourage me from crying. With anger, however, I was less self-supportive and I was not externally supported for this feeling at all.

Nurses walked out of the room if I began to talk about anger and all the psychiatrist said was, "You *should* feel angry. It's natural." This did nothing to support my *expression* of anger, however. Then one day Susan came.

Susan had been one of my former clients in my private practice. She herself was a very talented dancer and also a counselor with others. I felt like I needed her help in the worst way. "Please, Susan, you've got to help me with something," I pleaded.

"What's that, John?"

"I feel so full of rage. I know this is the second step of the grief process and that I should have it but I'm terrified of how much fury I feel. I'm scared of my own feelings. Help me to get some out."

"Sure." Susan first went and closed the door. She returned and bent down over the bed taking one of my pillows. "Here." She handed it to me with an instruction, "Just squeeze this with all your might and say whatever you need to say." I began squeezing on the pillow. Suddenly, the rage struck. A growl, low at first, began in the back of my throat. It rose both in pitch and intensity until I was expressing with my voice the incredible depth of rage that I felt. The loss. The horror. The sitting on the road, holding my own ragged leg in my hands. The pain. The fury. It all came rushing up. I strangled the pillow as I yelled about the unfairness of life. After only a minute or so the door swung open.

"What is going on here?" The nurse was red-faced and cross. "You are making too much noise." We explained to her what was happening. She told us it had to stop..."would stop immediately." I felt totally intimidated. I clamped down on my anger and felt a substitute feeling instead: terror. Susan was asked—told—to leave. Another nurse came into the room with the medication. Haldol. They would be certain that I didn't express anything else that I was feeling. The depression became a black pit with no bottom.

CHAPTER 3

They say that people's lives flash in front of them when they are going to die. During the first month and a half I spent in the hospital, I often felt like I might die. Sometimes I felt, odd as it may sound, as if I were already dead. Some part of me had died. I was now living some kind of "new life." During the day I didn't think a great deal about my "former life." I was able to keep myself preoccupied with one thing or another. I usually enjoyed visitors and could frequently distract myself quite well with them. At night I would fall into a semidrowsy state or even fall into a deep sleep, though I never dreamt—at least I had no awareness of ever dreaming (I suspect that all of the medication had something to do with preventing me from dreaming, but I'm not certain). I would often wake up in the middle of the night, however, and remember scenes from my life. Sometimes I would try to make a connection between these past events and what had happened to me in the accident. This kind of thinking was more like a search for meaning in the midst of a generally meaningless situation, an attempt to make sense in the face of a senseless event. Why had this happened to me? What must I have done in my life to make God, the Cosmos or Whatever-the-Heck do this to me? These were some of the questions that motivated my mental search into my past. I reviewed my life in compulsive detail to see what had gone wrong.

I had been born and raised in Derby, Connecticut. It was a tiny, industrial city of 13,000. My dad was a pin maker. He had worked for 42 years, sometimes for ten hours a day, six days a week, making common, ordinary straight pins. This job may sound simple and boring but Dad was like a Zen master of pin making. He was able to pick up a pin, roll it between his fingers and tell to within several thousandths of an inch what the diameter was or if the point was beveled at the correct angle. He was also quite handy and was able to fix almost anything that broke in the house, although he had absolutely no sense of aesthetics. If something worked, even if it looked really ugly, that was fine with him. He also made a lot of things for us. An orphan from the age of eight, Dad had a great deal of difficulty showing his feelings, so the things he made—a rose arbor for mom, a telescope mount for my brother Ernie, a lab table for me to do experiments on—these were his ways of telling us how much he cared for us.

Once, when Dad had fallen off of a ladder in the garage and tore a huge piece of flesh out of his shoulder, he had come into the house, got out the Mercurochrome and, sitting on the edge of the sink, proceeded to pour the vile liquid down the jagged wound in his back. He didn't make a sound or complain. Similarly, years later when he had cancer of the colon, stomach, and associated connective tissues, he would often sit for hours by the dining room table looking out the window at the street. He would never complain about the obvious pain he was in. It was, however, given away by the occasional involuntary grimaces and groans he would let out. We also saw him vomit huge quantities of blood and defecate blood with each bowel movement. He frequently had to go into the hospital, not for any treatment for the cancer or for any pain medication (he took none), but just to get transfusions to keep himself alive.

Dad and I did not have a particularly close relationship. He was hard of hearing from working around the old-fashioned, belt-driven machinery of the pin factory. We always had to yell at one another in order to have a conversation. This hearing problem made it rather difficult to have any kind of intimate exchange of feelings between us, except when dad was dying of cancer in 1976. He had never spoken of love to any of us throughout most of his life. About two weeks before he died, though, he leaned forward from his chair by the table, grabbed at his aching belly and said, "Johnny boy. I never told you this but I love you and your brother Ernie very much and I'm very proud of you both." Tears shot from my eyes. I had to rush from the room in order not to let him see how deeply overwhelmed I was by my own sudden awareness of the love I had for him all of these years. I was also eternally grateful to him that he made that effort to tell me of *his* love before he died. I have often looked back on that time as the one verbal affirmation of something that was evident in so many other ways nonverbally. I needed the verbal affirmation, however.

Dad was also quite stubborn. Once he set his mind to something, he usually stuck to it. I suspect that I got my stubborn ability to go on in the face of adversity from him. When I lay in bed in the hospital and thought about him, all I felt was missing him and wishing that we had spent more time together when I was a child. I certainly had done nothing toward my father for which I felt guilty, nothing that led me to believe that my accident was the result of any wrong-doing that I might have committed against him. How about my mother?

My mom was a housewife, mostly. She also liked to weave cloth and did that for Tingue Mills in Naugatuck, Connecticut until the hurricane of '56 wiped out the plant (and a great deal of the rest of the industrial "valley area"). She had studied opera from her teens until she met Richard. That was not the name of my father, but rather the man with whom Mom was madly in love before she had known Dad. Richard was also a singer, but regardless of Mom's intense feelings, he didn't show the slightest interest in her. She was crushed. So pained was she by the rejection that she decided to give up her voice training altogether. It was clearly an act of spite, and as in all such acts, her "nose" suffered.

After she married dad she became a full-time wife and mother, but I don't think she was ever truly happy without Richard and away from her chosen career. Mom was very emotional. Her ability to be empathic to others and her genuine concern for other people and living things was, I'm certain, at the foundation of my eventually going into the field of psychotherapy. She also taught me how to cry, thank God. This would save my life many times during the difficult years which would follow my becoming an adult. Unfortunately, Mom additionally taught me how to worry about almost anything. This last way of thinking was to become a great problem on my road to recovery from the accident but was clearly not the cause of it. I had no unfinished business with Mom that could have resulted in God's sending that truck to meet me on June 11th. How about my relationship to Ernie?

Ernie was my older brother—ten years older, to be exact. He was a scientist type and was always experimenting with something electrical or chemical. He was also my mentor—*a master*—(I did say in the ICU that I was studying with some sort of "master." What did that mean? I guess that I just wanted to return to the simple times when my brother pretty much guided the things I did, the projects that I would make. I wanted someone else to take over my life.) Ernie had taught me all kinds of wonderful things about science. I learned electricity, electronics, chemistry, astronomy, geology and numerous things about the physical sciences from him. He tutored me in amateur radio. Hours of time were spent on the theory and construction of radio circuitry. He started me on Morse Code and, although he himself did not apply for his license for many years, it was due to his diligent and thorough teaching that I was eventually able to pass the test for the F.C.C. Amateur Radio License at the Technician level.

He sponsored me to science fairs and prepared me for M.I.T. throughout my time in high school. He was my greatest hero as a child and we were always very close. When I thought of Ernie on some of those dark nights in the hospital, I had no reason to believe that anything that happened between us could be responsible for my "punishment." In fact, Ernie and I were almost always the best of friends. We literally had *no* sibling rivalry (he was so many years older that he was like another "father" to me) and, therefore, almost never fought.

I had a number of friends in high school, mostly around extracurricular activities. While I never played any school sports, I did enjoy being in the science club, the astronomical club, the debating team, the Yearbook staff, the literary magazine, the chess club, and the National Honor Society. I searched through my associations with each of my friends and, again, came up without a clue. We had fought like most people in relationships do, but we generally still loved one another, despite long distances and the passage of time.

Ed Santella was my all-time best friend. Ed and I met when our mothers were pushing us around in baby carriages. We grew up in adjacent yards, hung out together and played childhood games together. In high school Ed and I enjoyed shortwave radio and collecting the QSL cards which other countries sent for reports on their broadcasts. We were also active in astronomy, rock collecting, stamp collecting, and playing cards together. Whenever one or the other of us was concerned about something, we would get together to talk it over. Sometimes we did this while driving around in his old Chevy.

Eddie was always a bit more shy than I, but he turned out to be a lawyer after a stint in the Air Force (I always found both things incongruent with his personality, but he has done a good job as a lawyer). We truly loved each other and I had no troubling memories from my times with Ed. In fact, when I thought about the *people* of my childhood, I felt no particular guilt. There was an *event*, however, that did trouble me. When I remembered going off to college, something began to come back.

I had done pretty well in high school. I had won scads of honors and always kept up "A" grades. I got early acceptance to college and went off to M.I.T. to become a nuclear physicist. That's what my brother had become. Ernie was very self-directed; I was more of a "reactor." Anyway, I went to M.I.T. in my brother's footsteps, but unlike him, I got monumentally depressed. I found out that despite my lusty interest in science in high school, I didn't like nuclear physics at the college level. It was too cold for me. The classes were gigantic and impersonal. Several of my fellow freshmen committed suicide in the first year. I also got miserably homesick. I was raised to stay close to home.

My mother had taught me that the world was essentially a dangerous place (to worry about) and to stay at the house and study. Joe, a kid who had beaten me up frequently, reinforced the message. Being at home was great for learning. It allowed me to do what was necessary to get accepted to college. It was, however, totally inadequate at preparing me for independent life. It did not ready me for becoming a freshman in college, a hundred miles away from Derby.

Unable to concentrate or study, I had to drop out after only one semester, on "academic probation." It was very discouraging. I was *supposed* to be a nuclear physicist ever since I could remember. Even in the second grade I recall telling the teacher that I would be one when I grew up. I had to explain to her what a nuclear physicist did for a living but it was very thrilling being a kind of child prodigy to everyone. Maybe that was it? Maybe I violated my destiny to become a scientist? No—I had already paid painfully for that error of judgment. I had felt guilty about not completing M.I.T. for years and had eventually made up for my "failure."

Following that first terrible semester and my return home in disgrace, I went to the personnel department at Griffin Hospital to get a job as an orderly until I felt safe to try college again. When I got there and showed them my resume and my file of newspaper clippings, the people in personnel told me that I was "overqualified and should consider working in the laboratory." I went to interview with Dr. Dwight Miller, head of pathology.

He looked over my file. He read about my numerous academic and extracurricular achievements, furrowed his forehead and puffed out his breath. I thought that he seemed impressed.

"It looks like you've done quite a bit of research. Do you know anything about spectrophotometry?"

"Yes. I built a gamma ray spectrometer to measure the energy intensities of gamma particles from various radioactive sources for a science fair project." He looked quite interested, so I went on. "I also plotted energy spectra so that I could identify the source of the radiation as, for example, Strontium 90, etc."

"Well, we've got a Bausch and Lomb 505, dual-beam spectrophotometer in our new research lab and I would like someone to develop a series of tests to analyze a patient's blood to find unknown toxins. I would also like to be able to get a level for the toxin once identified by the U.V. spectrum. This would tell the ER people what they were dealing with if a patient came in comatose. Do you know what I'm talking about?"

"Yes. I do. When would you like me to begin?" I eagerly replied.

Six months later I completed my work as chief researcher for the laboratory of Griffin Hospital. I published the results through Yale and returned to college, this time at Fairfield University, to study pre-medicine. I thought I might want to become a doctor. I never did go on to medical school, however. Did I fail there? Maybe I should have become a doctor?

"I don't know. I just don't fucking know." I said to myself in the hospital bed. After all, wasn't I now in a doctoral program? Hadn't I almost finished with the research for my doctoral dissertation by the summer of 1981? I had proven to my family *and* to myself that I could be successful academically. Was there something else that I was guilty of? My mind wandered on, relentlessly, restlessly, blamefully, searching for the answer to a question of meaning.

In July I was moved to White Plains Hospital to undergo skin graft surgery on the denuded right foot.

CHAPTER 4

The two burly EMTs gently lifted the stretcher from the hospital emergency bay entrance into the back of the ambulance. I guess they were trying not to shake me up, but they weren't succeeding. I was obviously in considerable pain from the pins through my leg, but I was being pretty good (again) about the transport. I just lay there staring straight ahead at the traction apparatus that was attached to the Hoffman frame on my right foot. The foot wobbled back and forth like a wrecking ball on a crane as the stretcher was locked into place. I remember letting out one muffled groan. "Don't drop the fucking weights or I'll deck you bastards," I thought. I kept watching the weights swinging back and forth. Each movement sent a pulling, burning sensation through my leg as six metal pins tugged against nerve endings. The Dilaudid they gave me for the transport wasn't doing the trick. I still felt every jerk, every fast movement. I thought I'd go through the roof when one fellow bumped the traction pole. After mentally cursing him, I just returned to staring at the cables and their five-pound weights.

There was a nurse on the platform of the Emergency Room entrance. Her uniform was nice, clean and white. My right foot was cloaked in nice, clean, white bandages. As she turned to go back into the Emergency Room, I thought about how strange the procedure must have been. Another nurse on the afternoon shift told me about it. The doctors had to wrap my foot in living animal tissue. "Oh well," she had told me, "using porcine skin is probably an important step in keeping the subdermis from drying out. I never heard of this procedure, but I'm sure it's the right thing to do." I wondered how she would have felt with the skin of a pig wrapped around her leg.

"Pig skin," I thought. "I feel like some goddamn, composite laboratory experiment." My left leg was missing, covered by a cast and my right foot was part pig. *I* was part *pig* for God's sake!

Both EMTs were quite friendly. They tried to talk to me about the ambulance, what they did on a typical day and what they thought about transports. I really had a difficult time concentrating on what they were saying, however. I felt only partially there. I think that my answers were coherent, but I was clearly distracted. Mostly, my mind was occupied by thoughts of happier times.

"...So there was this one transport when we forgot to lock the wheelchair in and during the ride the old lady was cursing at us from the back. When I checked...." His voice drifted off into oblivion. I went back inside of myself again. A sadness of gigantic proportions began to well up in my chest. I choked back the tears. I saw myself standing on a modeling stand at Silvermine Guild for Artists. I thought, "I used to be able to maintain without motion the most difficult poses for twenty minutes easily. I especially loved the one where I crossed my feet...now there's only one foot...in what in Karate is called the 'Hook Stance.' My arms arranged on the diagonal, curved from shoulder to finger tip, head tilted to one side. What an artistic challenge to sketch. What a beautifully creative gesture to make with my body." The hot tears were now coming in streams down my cheeks.

"When I checked..." he said.

"Yeah," I nodded. I was being polite, but I wasn't really listening. I felt so absorbed in my own loss and...fear! I was going *away* from Danbury Hospital. I had just begun to adjust to the idea of being in the hospital at one location, and now I was going somewhere else. It would be farther away. I wouldn't know anyone. Carolyn would have a harder time getting to see me. God, how I missed her. I began to cry again at this new thought.

The surgery at White Plains consisted of using a machine called a dermatome to literally shave off outer layers of skin in strips two inches wide by fourteen inches long. The entire skin cover of the right thigh was removed. The newly denuded dermis filled with nerve endings was covered with Opcite, a kind of giant, plastic, adhesive tape that would remain in place until the new skin grew out. The Opcite would then, according to the physician in charge, "simply be peeled off without discomfort." The right foot had to be stripped of porcine skin and be scraped up so that it would have a bleeding, living area of tissue, receptive to the skin grafts. This was all done under total anesthetic, of course, so that I would be spared any unnecessary trauma or pain.

Dr. Robert Reiffel bent over the bottom end of my bed. He was absorbed in thought as he slowly peeled away the layers of moistened gauze from the grafted skin. "Just hold on, John," he muttered. "I'm sorry to hurt you but I'm almost done with this layer." I began sobbing now as the tweezers passed between two skin edges and nicked the exposed nerve endings on the front of the foot. A little blood began to run from the area. The nurse leaned forward and dabbed at the trickle with a 4″ × 4″ pad. The last layer of gauze was tough. No amount of soaking could loosen the glue made by the serosanguinous ooze. "This is going to hurt more," he said matter-of-factly and he began the task of tearing off the adhering bandage. More sobbing was heard. Now and again I gave out an even louder groan. Finally, after another half hour, I leaned forward and waved my hands in the air.

"Stop it, goddamn it. I can't take it any more," I wailed. "Please, I'm begging you, please give me something for the pain."

Reiffel looked me in the eye. It seemed as though an understanding surpassing the words flashed between us.

"Nurse, get me Valium I.V. and Dilaudid I.V." He would give this order each time there was to be a dressing change.

The nurse returned with the two syringes. Reiffel picked them both up and came around to the left side of the bed. He lay one of them down, tied a rubber tourniquet around my arm above the elbow and palpating the brachial vein, wiped the area clean with an alcohol wipe and slid the needle easily into the ropey tube. Within a few minutes I slipped into a dark, peaceful sleep. They could work more rapidly then.

Thirty-two days I had spent in Danbury Hospital, and now I was to spend at least another month at White Plains. I had lain flat on my back every minute. There was no respite. During the day I would hunger for visitors. I would exhaust myself with them, trying to escape the horror of my existence and my losses. I had been given plenty of crossword puzzles and greeting cards. At least a dozen of my relatives were having Masses said for me—religious orders I had never even heard of in some cases.

One person whom I could have strangled brought me a new mechanical puzzle that was taking the country by storm. It was called a Rubic's Cube and it was made by the Devil himself. When I first got it I was able to rotate one section 180 degrees and return it to its original position, preserving the completed cube. After a few more tries I got braver and rotated several sections 180 degrees. Well, that was the end of order and the beginning of chaos. I suppose there might be people with functioning brains who could actually derive pleasure out of attempting to solve such a riddle, but for my depressed mind it was only one more impossible frustration to contend with. I was still stuck in a deep melancholy and I was feeling more and more disconsolate as each day went by.

There were the dressing changes on a regular basis. I actually welcomed them because I would be put to sleep and could escape everything at least for an hour or so. Mealtime was still an adventure in "time-passing." It didn't matter how tasteless the food was, the hospital meal was a welcome interruption to an otherwise pointless existence. I finally resolved that I had to do something with my depressed feelings and began to search for a nurse who might help me facilitate my unfelt anger (remembering the incident with Susan). It was on an afternoon shift that I met Selma, a nursing supervisor.

Selma was a large, jovial black woman who told me that she had a great deal of training in psychiatric nursing and that she would be happy to help me deal with the anger that I was feeling..."to get it *out*." I recollected to her all of the difficulties I had experienced with the professional staff around my angry feelings. She showed a great deal of empathy and told me, "Hospitals just are not that sensitive to the emotional needs of the patients they seek to help. But...well...the body needs a healthy mind to help it heal." She smiled and I nodded in agreement. We planned to meet on the following Wednesday, sometime in the afternoon.

I awoke that Wednesday in July actually feeling a bit hopeful. Today I would begin to get some relief from the gnawing rage that was all turned back at myself. I waited anxiously throughout the morning and hardly touched the lunch. At 1:00 o'clock I started looking at one of the comic books which one visitor had the good sense to bring me. It was all I had the mental ability to comprehend. By 2:00 o'clock I had inspected every mindless picture in the entire assortment. I began drawing in a pad at 2:30. By 3:00 I had done several dozen doodles. None of them looked like anything. I wasn't able to complete any kind of complex picture. 3:30, 3:45, 3:50, 3:55, 3:56, and thirty seconds went by. I was now doing nothing but watching the large round clock on the wall opposite to my bed. This was no good. I had to find some way to pass time until the cavalry came. I saw the television screen. "Soap operas" was what came immediately to mind. I decided to see what was on anyway. I turned on the T.V. Every channel available was showing a soap. It was after 4:00 p.m., so the story was already in progress—not that that mattered with a soap. I changed from program to program. The stories were mostly the same: "somebody's lover was pregnant with the baby of the married friend in the next apartment and she was worried about having an abortion." There was also: "Bill is dying in the hospital and must try to gain the forgiveness of his friend with whose wife he has been having an affair for the past eight years."

When I was finished it was 5:00 p.m. Wasn't the afternoon over? Didn't afternoons have a limit to them, like around 5:00 p.m. or so? I was accustomed to waiting for doctors. I had waited once five days for a doctor to come in to see me at Danbury. I was so spaced out on drugs there that the waiting was tolerable, however. Here I was more lucid. I counted minutes in *this* hospital room and there was something unimaginably aggravating about having to lay in one position for more than forty days just so I could wait minute by minute for a psychiatric nurse who would help me get to feeling some emotional relief. At 6:03 p.m. the food cart arrived. The smell of very over-cooked victuals wafted together into an indescribable food-o-montage. It didn't matter. That smell marked a wonderful way to pass time. I would be pleasantly occupied for at least the next hour—not that it took an hour to eat what I was given. It was the way that I ate that drew out this otherwise uneventful activity into the best occupational therapy anyone could ever hope for in the hospital.

I always began by first surveying the tray. I received this one by 6:27 and greeted it by lifting the large stainless steel steam cover off of the dinner plate. There was a hole in the top in which I could insert my finger. I didn't know if it was intended for this purpose. The hole served as an escape for the steam and sometimes the hot air rushed past my digits as I raised the cover off of the dish. I carefully looked for a place on the tray where I could place the cover without occluding my view of anything else I had been brought. "Ah, there is the carton of milk," I thought with a strange and vague sense of pleasure. I pulled the lip forward on one side and poured it into the glass.

Each day there was a ritual of making out a "menu"—a chance to select one of four possible dishes for dinner. I always forgot what I had picked. Tonight it was fish. Too bad. If it had been chicken I could spend the longest time using a knife and fork to dissect the meat from the bones. I could go after every tiny morsel with the fork tines, shave fat from the back of the skin with the edge of the knife blade. But tonight I would just have to chew the fish filet extra slowly—Fletcherize it. Along with the fish there were green peas and mashed potatoes. The potatoes were instant, of course, but that was O.K. One doesn't really have a keen sense of flavor when depressed, anyway. Besides, the kitchen had remembered to include the salt and pepper packets, so I could spend a few moments dressing up the potatoes before eating them with a spoon in small mouthfuls. Using different utensils passed time as well. There was the activity of putting down the fork so I could pick up the spoon, etc.

There was a bit of paprika on the fish. It didn't really make the food more appetizing, but I did notice it. I next went through the act of putting the butter onto the peas. They were already cool and the butter (already mushy) just sat there. I salted and peppered the potatoes and placed the empty paper packets back into the paper cup in which they had come. Unfolding the napkin, I tucked it into the collar of my white "johnny coat," smoothed it out, and then reached for my utensils. I liquified each bite of food. It wasn't hot and it wasn't delicious, but it was important to the passage of time. I lay down the knife and fork between each bite so that I could take a sip of the milk. I could always muster enough concentration to deal with this primitive feeding activity. When I was finished, the plate would be completely wiped clean of any clue that it once held food. This latter act was effected by the careful use of the single slice of white bread which was included with each dinner if I bothered to select it on the menu earlier. I always did. The bread came snuggled in Saran wrap. It usually took a while to unwrap it and, if I had another piece of butter, to spread with the mushy, yellow paste. I had wiped the plate clean in bits, tearing off pieces of the buttered bread and skating them each around a different, small part of the plate. There was some mushy butter left from the peas. There was also some mashed potatoes and a tiny puddle of juice from the fish filet. The swabbing acts completed, it was then possible for me to begin a whole new ritual with the dessert. That day it was cling peaches in a small, pink, plastic dish. I carefully lifted the dish and with my spoon cut a bite-sized piece off of each slice of peach. Eventually and with some regret I lifted the Melamine dish to my lips to sip down the watery syrup that lay in the bottom. There! The meal was finished. Time?

"7:24 p.m. Almost an hour!" I mumbled out loud.

Where the hell was Selma? Surely afternoon had passed! Was I being stood up? Was she afraid of my anger? I was.

Evening television helped to pass a great deal of time. I wasn't able to understand much of the more complex shows. The police and other violent shows scared me (I was too afraid of my own anger and rage). I was reduced to watching sitcoms. My depression made the shows unfunny but they were always an opportunity to watch a constantly changing series of visual images that were not threatening in any way. Finally it was 10:00 p.m. I wasn't tired. I was emotionally exhausted! But I also felt agitated. I would have trouble sleeping again tonight. My body was healing. I was more energized and had no way to tire myself during the day. I lay in bed—the *same* position I had been in for over a month—thinking about Selma. I was too depressed to strongly dislike her but I didn't feel any better that she hadn't shown. At 11:15 Selma arrived.

"Hi. I'm here just like I said I would be." Inappropriately bright and cheerful, she entered the room.

"Where were you? I have been waiting all day for you to come." There was a little bit of irritation in my voice, but there was more disappointment.

"Oh...didn't I tell you? My shift had been changed."

"No! You didn't tell me." The "no", this time, had some expression in it but the rest of the statement sounded flat and unemotional. I felt flat. My feelings were slipping away more and more easily. "Please! I need to express a lot of anger and I want to be able to release it, but I am aware that it is so late that most of the other patients are asleep right now. What do I do?"

"Well, I'll just sit here..."—she pulled up a yellow armchair—"...and you can talk out your anger to me."

"Talk out? Don't you know that talking *about* angry subjects in a calm voice only makes a person more depressed? I need to talk *in an angry way*!"

"O.K. You do what you have to."

The look in her eyes was one of confidence and self-assuredness. I trusted and believed her. I then remembered the sand bag. I took the black, leather bag filled with sand that the occupational therapist had brought me several days ago in order to exercise my arms. I placed it on the bed to my right side but away from the raw areas of unhealed skin. While I spoke of my resentment about having so much taken away from me in the accident I made emphatic hits on the bag (a way to act out in the body the anger that needed expression, much like a speaker makes his point by hitting the top of the podium). As soon as I started, Selma interrupted.

"Now, now. You have to calm down. Try to be reasonable about all this. If you're going to go hitting things then I'm going to have to leave."

I felt like she had just slapped my face. I lay there benumbed. The critical control mechanism in my brain took over and I plummeted into more depression and flatness. "I'm not angry anymore," I said, lying. I hoped that at least I wouldn't be abandoned by her now as well.

"O.K. Good. I've got other things to tend to. See you later." And with that she got up and left. I stayed awake that night.

One day a strange thing happened: Burke came to the door. I had heard that there was another patient on the ward who was approximately my age, and I had wanted desperately to meet him. Well, here he was. He wasn't much to look at, unshaven, unkempt, with his leg up in a cast covered with food droppings and dirt. But there he was in his wheelchair just like my nurse had promised.

"Hi there."

"Hi," I returned. "God, but it's good to see you."

"Why the hell would it be good to see me?" He retorted with a shrug.

"Because I've been so fucking lonely here, that's why. The nurses are good to look at and all that...." He smiled and nodded at that statement.

"But...I have just wanted to hang out with someone. They told me you were here. I'm John."

"Yeah, John. Well I'm Burke. What you got?"

"I was in an accident and I lost my leg. How about you?"

"Osteo."

"Huh. What's that?"

"It's a bone infection. I was a vet in Nam. I got hit by shrapnel from a Claymore and I was patched up at a M.A.S.H. unit. They thought I was all healed up and sent me back into action but when I got stateside I found out I had this stuff called osteomyelitis."

"You going to be O.K.?"

"I don't know. After I got shot up in the war I got all bummed out and...hey...have you done your 'sick shit' yet?"

"Maybe. What's 'sick shit'?"

"You know. That's when you get all pissed off and start throwing food trays around and tell the nurses to 'fuck off' and all that stuff that has to do with losing your leg."

I just lay there and marveled at him. An ex-marine was telling me, a psychotherapist, what I needed to do psychotherapeutically. The damned thing was that he was absolutely right. "Nope. Not yet."

"Well," he said, simultaneously turning his right wheel forward and his left wheel backward so that he was aimed toward the open door. "Let me know when you do. You'll be worth talking to then." And then he just...left!

When I saw the door close I knew that I had to get through my "sick shit" more than ever. This Vietnam vet impressed me. He said what I had been thinking all along: that I needed to experience my anger fully and with self-acceptance. I couldn't yell at the nurses or throw things at them, they were too nice. In fact, they were disgustingly polite. Every morning a nurse would bounce cheerfully into the room and call out, "Good morning. How are we this morning?" or something equivalent. Once, when a friend, John Mickelson, came to visit me he asked me what I wanted. I said, "I'd like a nurse to come into my room just once and say, 'Hey asshole, how come you didn't lose the other one?' Then I could get justifiably pissed at her." With this wish unlikely to be fulfilled, I would have to take care of myself.

I began working out each day on my pillow and on the black, sand-filled bag I mentioned earlier. I spent at least an hour each day pounding and pounding. When I needed to scream out my rage, I would cover my mouth with several pillows and scream into them. On one occasion, looking down at the metal cage that surrounded my right foot, I saw myself as part man, part contraption and began to growl. The growling and snarling made me remember a Frankenstein movie I'd seen as a child, and I began to change the vocalizations into the sounds that the Frankenstein monster made. I ended up laughing that day. Throughout all of my personal work on anger no one ever came to my room or interfered with me. I guess that I had found a way to make noise into pillows well enough so that no one could hear me. I was safe to express myself now. One day when the rage hit with full force, I clobbered the pillow until it was completely shredded into pieces. When I was finished, I lay back in a puddle of my own sweat. Foam stuffing was all over the bed. I felt exhausted and relaxed. God, that was satisfying! No one asked me how the pillow got ripped up.

Two days later, I requested for Burke to come back. Within an hour he was shoving his wheelchair through my hospital room door. He wasn't in the room five minutes when he remarked, "Man, do you look different. Your face seems...I don't know...not so wacky. You've got some color, too. Have you been beating up on the nurses or something?"

"Nope. I have been 'spitting nails,' but mostly to myself. I feel a whole lot better, though."

"Good enough! So what's up with you...where you from anyway?..." He stayed for a long time that day and came back often.

Burke turned out to be a good friend to me and an excellent "buddy" with whom to hang out for a couple of hours every other day or so. We usually ended up talking about his Vietnam experiences. Apparently, Burke had been an assassin for Special Forces. He was sent on CIA organized missions, he said, into enemy areas to kill important military leaders and Viet Cong operatives in Saigon. I often found his stories a combination of fascinating, unbelievable, and frightening.

Since Burke was the one who was mobile, I had to depend mostly upon his schedule and mobility to get together with him. Sometimes his legs hurt so badly he wouldn't go out in the chair, and on other days when I would ask for him, he'd be off in some other part of the hospital for treatments or physical therapy. After only two weeks of this relationship, Burke disappeared. I was told he was discharged. He never came to say goodbye. I was sad about that. "Other men are so emotionally insensitive," I thought. I heard the voices of many women with whom I had worked over the years as they said the same thing.

While Bob Reiffel was officially my doctor throughout my stay at White Plains, his associate often came in to examine the dressing and to see to it that the pin sites on the Hoffman had not become infected. I forget his name these many years later, but I shall never forget how he made his entrance. He would walk directly toward the right side of the bed where my foot was held by the traction apparatus. As he did so his gaze was fixed intently on the metal configuration as if to avert his vision might be a violation of the Hypocratic oath. When he arrived at the side of the bed he always bent forward to inspect the traversing rods more closely and always struck the top of his head on the trapeze frame above the bed. He would then vocalize his discomfort, "Ouch!", rub his head, and proceed to poke around the bandages and dressings. This must have happened at least a dozen times in the month that I was there and I unremittingly found it amusing and entertaining. I entitled it, "Moe (of Three Stooges fame) becomes a doctor." My seeing the humor in this event was a distinct sign of my own mental recovery. There was still, however, a great deal more to do.

Each day nurses came and went in and out of Room 206. It was necessary to change my dressings, bring and remove bedpans, change the bed, perform "pin care" (cleaning the rods that went through both sides of the right shin and the heelbone), and to remove the empty bag of antibiotic solution that constantly dripped into my arm. The antibiotics were very important. All possible infectants had to be arrested early on. So far, my body had responded well and I didn't have so much as a cold.

The bag-changing procedure was pretty much the same each day. The nurse would come over to the left side of my bed where the IV pole was set up, reach up to the plastic line that entered the bag, and close the rollerlock. This device pinched off the tube when the sharpened cannula was pulled out of the old bag and inserted into the full one. Lastly, the nurse had to hang the new plastic bag onto the hook at the top of the metal pole, undo the rollerlock and reestablish the correct flow of drops per minute for that particular fluid and the particular patient. On July 18th my fluid bags were changed several times during the day. One more change would occur during the night.

A Jamaican-born nurse apparently took the orders for medications for her shift that night. I imagine that she saw that the "skin graft" would need a change of antibiotics. She must have gone to the drug cart where these fluids were prepared fresh daily by the in-house pharmacy and selected the correct solution for her patient. When she entered the room at approximately 4:00 a.m., she had to turn on a cantilevered lamp attached to the wall to the left of the bed. If she wanted to keep from waking me up she would have had to quickly point the hood opening away from the bed. She may have attempted the maneuver, but it was too late. When the light went on, I moved restlessly and opened my eyes. I don't remember saying anything, but I'm sure that I gave off a grunt in response to the interruption of sleep. I then proceeded to watch the clear, plastic tube in front of me. My eyes began to focus through the fog. Somewhere in my awakening brain I knew what was happening. I perceived that this was a routine procedure and nothing to be concerned about, but I was awake then. I watched the plastic tube that dangled and twisted as the nurse removed the cannula. The tube lifted slightly as she temporarily hung it over the top of the IV pole. The swinging slowed and the tube almost came to rest when something caught my eye. It was the meniscus, the curved shape that liquid makes when it approaches the edges of the container that holds it. The meniscus was sliding down the tube at an incredible rate. I opened my eyes wider as I followed the surface of the antibiotic liquid to the white tape holding the needle in the vein.

"Hmmm," I thought without emotion. "There goes the last of the stuff into my arm. Now there's air going into my arm."

I had not moved yet. Then, after a few more moments, I felt the flutter in my chest...in my heart! I sat bolt upright in the bed and instinctively grabbed the tubing, folded it over, and held it closed.

"What the hell are you doing?" I demanded. "You are putting air into my veins, goddamn you!"

The nurse seemed totally shocked. "I dun knoh wut you soo upset. Dere's nutting be wurried abut."

"Air!! Don't you understand? You are putting air into me. You forgot to close the rollerlock on the hose!" Sure enough, the lock was still open. "Get me the night supervisor right now!" I yelled.

"Dun wurry. Nutting bad wud happen to you."

"And make sure she speaks English!"

The nurse hesitated for a moment at this last insult and then ran from the room, dropping the empty plastic bag she had been holding in her hand.

Within minutes an older and very professional nurse entered the room. "Mr. Gagnon?" I nodded. "Mrs. Shantamon tells me that you are upset about something...a mistake?"

"Upset? Upset? Of course I'm upset!" I was practically hysterical now. "Do you see this tubing here? Well, I'm closing it off right now with my hand. If I wasn't holding it closed there would be air flowing steadily into my vein. I could die from this mistake!"

"Now Mr. Gagnon," she said in a tone that a mother would use with a foolish child. She shook her head in contrived frustration and then walked over to the left side of the bed and contemplated and closed the valve. "I'm sure that you could not have received any more than a few cc's of air. That would be perfectly harmless. Nothing would have happened to you. I'm sure the nurse would have hung the other bag and reconnected the tubing before there was any problem." Her face wore a plastic smile.

"I *felt* the air in my *heart*! Don't you get it? If she had gone back to the nurse's station because she had forgotten something I could have been lying here for minutes, pumping enough cc's of air to stop my heart with an embolus."

Again the chiding voice spoke. "I think you are distraught, Mr. Gagnon.

I don't think that anything *that* serious would have happened. O.K.?"

"No! It's not O.K. I want to speak to my doctor in the morning. I want to file a formal complaint."

"Well...I'm the night supervisor and *I* will file the complaint for you."

"You can file whatever you like. I will still complain and...I want to see my doctor in the morning, understood?"

"Yes. Now you just rest easily while Mrs. Shantamon hangs up the new antibiotic. O.K.?"

"The hell I will. You get some other nurse in here to do that." Then, realizing my need for a more authoritative sound to this statement, I added, "She *does not have my permission to perform that procedure*..." and sarcastically amended, "O.K.?"

"All right, all right, if you insist I'll ask Karen to come in. Is that all right?"

Thinking first about who Karen was, I replied, "Yes. That'll be fine. Thank-you!"

Turning on her white, rippled shoes with a squeak she concluded the conversation. "Goodnight, Mr. Gagnon. You get some rest now."

There was no rest for nearly a week. The doctor had said that it would have taken at least 10 cc's to kill someone. That didn't seem correct. I remembered that doctors in the past had always squirted some of the liquid out of the syringe to get rid of, I thought, the tiniest bit of air. I really felt paranoid now. The people into whose hands I had placed myself for care could have killed me. It also didn't help to have visitors come in with horror stories that heightened my paranoia.

Betty listened to me tell her about the IV.

"That's nothing," she said, smoothing the front of her skirt. "My uncle was in the hospital in '78 for a gall bladder problem. They made some kind of mistake....I don't remember what it was now...anyway they gave him a massive infection. By the time they got it cleared up, both his kidneys were shot. He was on dialysis for a whole year before he died."

"Charming...just charming!" I thought. "Why the hell is she telling me this when I just said that I didn't trust the hospital staff?"

"That's too bad," I quipped, feeling a bit nauseous.

I was also able to recall times when I had seen mistakes made in hospitals in which I had worked. I once saw a man brought in with a heart attack. He was talking to me in the hallway before they got him into the emergency room. He coded en route and they decided at that moment that they would call him DOA. I remember yelling at the staff that I had just spoken to him and that he should be worked on. They ignored me and said that they were too busy. Recollections like this, the horror stories others continually told me, and my own experience with the IV were enough to keep me well frightened.

I don't think I slept at all for six or seven days. After that I could only doze restlessly. I felt pessimistic again, scared and depressed. I didn't feel in control of my life or of my own safety, and I couldn't really trust the hospital. I wanted some control.

One evening I had watched some television before retiring. *Evita*, the Broadway musical, was very popular at the time and it was being advertised in almost every break of Monday Night at the Movies. I finally dozed off around 2 or 3 a.m. and had a dream. It was about the stage production of *Evita*. I couldn't see any of the actors but I was certain that it was that particular play. I was not an actor in the play nor was I even a part of the backstage crew. I was the curtains! My job was to move the counter balances up and down (the traction apparatus at the foot of my bed at which I had stared for nearly two months) and make the curtains open and close. I controlled the curtains at least. It was all I would ever do, but in the dream I felt like I had to do my job well!

"It's time to change your IV" she said turning on the flexible lamp next to the bed.

"Is this *Evita*?" I pleaded for an answer.

"What?" The nurse looked completely confused.

"Is this the play, *Evita*...you know...the *play*!"

"No. You are in White Plains Hospital."

The fog began to part as my fears were once again realized. I knew where I was. I understood, sadly, that I was lying in a hospital bed. "I'm sorry...I am not making any sense," I uttered with tears in my eyes as the reality dawned in on me like the lamp light that had cut through my slumber. I cried myself back to sleep that night wishing that I was the curtains in the play, *Evita*.

CHAPTER 5

Many more restless nights came and went. I was still waking up and wondering, in some irrational way, what the possible cosmic cause of my suffering might be. "Why do bad things happen to good people?" I queried in my mind. "Maybe I'm not a good person," I lamented to myself in return. This might have been comforting in a perverse way if only I could find the incident(s) where I might have been such an unethical individual. The old business about college returned. I thought I had finished with this but evidently I had not. I thought, "Maybe this has something to do with my giving up on M.I.T.—not returning—switching majors and going to a different school? Maybe I should have stuck it out at M.I.T. regardless of how frightened I was? Maybe I should not have gone to Fairfield University to study premed?"

Fairfield was a good experience, actually. Not because it prepared me for medical school—I didn't study much about human anatomy or physiology in the undergraduate program called premedicine. While I was in the program, however, I did learn something much more valuable. What I learned was the Jesuit interpretation and presentation of Catholic theology.

We all had to take a certain number of theology courses in those days regardless of major. It was like a required minor in religious studies. In Fairfield University, I began to reassess my religious upbringing and, for the first time in my dogmatically prescribed life, to question a great deal about my religion. I found that the Jesuits were quite liberal in their thinking and that the concept of a Higher Power, sometimes referred to as God, could encompass a much more personal and loving existence than I had been raised to believe. The God of my youth was mostly punitive and frightening. I had been born and raised "old-time" Roman Catholic.

During the college years, I worked summers to help pay for tuition and board. The first job I had was for Central Guard Service in New Haven. It paid minimum wage, but I was often able to do a lot of reading and studying on certain guard assignments. I also worked for Pinkerton Detective Agency as a private investigator and for St. Vincent's Hospital in the general laboratory as a technician. In my junior year I added laboratory technician for the biology department to my job duties and also joined the Derby Police Department as an auxiliary officer and then a "special" (part-time officer). Apart from earning college costs, I was also searching for what I wanted to become throughout most of my stay at Fairfield.

It had become so difficult to find myself after I had given up a ten-year dream of becoming a nuclear physicist. I knew that I wanted to be in some kind of social service field, working with people or working to help people, but I still couldn't figure out what that was. With these doubts in my mind I wasn't yet ready to commit myself to medical school. Of that, at least, I was certain.

I had met a girl in my freshman year at Fairfield. Sharon and I dated for four years steadily, and when senior year rolled around, we got married. I was twenty-one and she was twenty. We were deeply in love. I wanted to work and make money and settle down. Medical school, *if* I decided to go there, could wait. Furthermore, I was tired of studying major subjects in which I had so little career interest. It was also 1969.

That was an important year to graduate from college. The draft was on and I needed to work at something that would keep me deferred. Don't misunderstand me. I really *was* opposed to the war in Vietnam. But I also didn't want to get hurt or killed. Just the thought of being hurt made me want to "run back home" again like I did from M.I.T.

I finally located a nice, draft-deferred teaching post at Nathan Hale Junior High School in New Britain, Connecticut with a shared-time position at St. Ann's Junior High School one block over. I became a seventh-, eighth- and ninth-grade science teacher. It was quite different for me at first, but after a while I learned to love the children and hate the job. Teaching was just not right for me. The best part of my work was staying after to help some kid who was struggling with a peer or home problem. I liked counseling my students. As the months turned into years I realized that I had not yet actually chosen my own career or a vocation toward which I might turn my energies with interest. I felt pressured to make a career decision soon. My early life experience as a Roman

Catholic and my courses in theology at Fairfield helped me to make that decision. I knew that I wanted to work in a field that would allow me to be involved with people. I wanted to be a helper in some way. Serving others in a spiritual way *might be* what I was looking for.

Since moving to New Britain to teach I had attended the Church of Divine Light in Hartford where I went twice each week to study religious, spiritual, and philosophical topics. We covered a wide range of world religions like Buddhism, Islam, Hinduism, various pentecostal movements, Taoism and even the ancient teachings of Zoroaster, and the writings of Hermes Trismagistus. For the first time in my life I had the opportunity to study a vast number of philosophical and theological perspectives from which to examine human existence within a spiritual framework.

I reexamined my early Catholic upbringing with such a fervor as to become thoroughly engrossed with religion during much of my free time. Each week members of the church would hold a forum to argue and discuss their understandings of one or more philosophical or theological points. I loved the intellectual exchange and stimulation. I began to formulate and evolve my own sense that there was Divine Truth, not in any one, single, organized religion but that there might be profound Truth in a unified theosophy which sought to integrate those fundamental essences or archetypal visions shared by all of them. I wanted to find a church in which all religions might be integrated and embraced as important. I was also looking for any organized religion that had a broader and more inclusive view of the God-Head or Cosmic Force or Prime Mover or whatever that transcendent spiritual power in life might be called. I found some of this in the Church of Divine Light, but they were clearly oriented more toward pentacostal applications of world-religion teachings: hands-on healing, spiritualism, etc. This was a little too "far out" for me. I wanted a more rational approach.

In the meantime, one of the members of that Hartford church had just become an ordained clergy-woman. I asked her how this was done since she had not been attending a seminary or divinity school. She told me that this was "a new time in the history of religion" and that if one was suitable to lead others in the pursuit of religious truth that there were religions which ordained persons based upon their sincerity, their pursuit of knowledge and their strength of "calling." The notion was completely new to me. I felt intrigued. After several months I asked her how I might find out more about this kind of church, and she simply referred me to an advertisement in a magazine. This ad offered ordination for those with a "spiritual calling." The more I thought about it, the more the idea of serving people in a spiritual way appealed to me. I had a genuine calling to that and to the varieties of religious experience. It had been born out by the zeal with which I had independently studied so much theology over the years. I wrote to them. After a brief correspondence, and with a clear understanding of the career into which I was about to embark, I accepted ordination as a minister of the Life Science Church.

I then studied even more intensely than before to make up for what I had not gotten in a seminary or divinity school. When I felt ready, I gathered together a congregation in New Britain. This new church took the name The Unified Church of the Divinity (of the Life Science Churches). I left teaching, pastored my congregation, became a member of the New Britain Clergy Association, and our church was made a member church of the New Britain Area Conference of Churches. I found myself truly happy. I was doing exactly what I had wanted to do most of my life, but now I could identify it. I enjoyed preaching, hospital visitation, and I especially enjoyed counseling persons in spiritual difficulty.

When I was lying in the hospital in 1981, however, I did not find any comfort in my understanding of God. I felt betrayed by Him. I couldn't comprehend why He would let this happen or do such a terrible thing to me. I was angry with my God for the pain he either caused others to have or allowed others to have. I was surrounded by reminders of this pain in the cries other patients made throughout the day and occasionally at night. Something about this remembering was helping me to get a handle, however, on what was torturing me emotionally, so I knew that I had to examine it more closely.

While in the New Britain Area Conference of Churches I met pastors of many diverse belief systems, and I was surprised to find a religion that was precisely like what I had been looking for: Unitarian Universalism. I enjoyed talking with Unitarians and found that I shared with them a common interest in religious exploration. As a result, I was invited to be a guest pastor at a number of Unitarian churches throughout Connecticut.

Applying myself to my career, in addition to my continuing duties as pastor, I offered my services to the New Britain Memorial Hospital where I became the chaplain to their patients, most of whom had chronic illnesses like muscular dystrophy or cerebral palsy. I ran a wide range of programs for the patients, counseled them and had local college professors come in to teach a philosophy course to them. Sharon and I were both happy with my chosen work and life was good and rich. There was an additional bonus as well.

As a Catholic it had been impossible for me to find forgiveness for myself. Forgiveness only took place through a priest. I often felt guilty as a child just for having thoughts that were considered "sinful" by the priests and nuns who taught me. Since I had become a minister (priest) I felt like I could release myself from the chains of guilt with which those early teachers had imprisoned me. My almost constant dread from childhood that I was "wrong" or "bad" vanished. I didn't understand this at the time, but for this and all of the joy I had received studying theology and being of service to others I was truly happy.

As I lay in my hospital bed in 1981 and thought about Catholicism and being a minister, something began to click about guilt. Was I punished for having become a minister? Should I have stayed in the Catholic Church as my mother had wanted? No, that didn't seem right. But in some way I knew that Catholicism did have some relationship to what I was feeling about my accident. What that relationship was I had no idea. "Anyway," I thought one day, "I don't believe in that dogmatic stuff anymore." I believed that I had left my old guilt-ridden youth behind. The search for an answer continued.

When I was a chaplain at New Britain Memorial Hospital, a Doctor Ill (I kid you not) suggested that I get more experience in counseling patients and recommended my applying to the Connecticut Valley Hospital School of Pastoral Care for training. I did and was accepted into this program in June of 1972.

I was tremendously impressed by my new instructors. They were caring and concerned about people and were also concerned mentors. This was a lot like returning to the kind of relationship I had enjoyed with my brother. It was one, I was to sadly discover later in my life, that was seldom if ever found in the work place.

At Connecticut Valley Hospital I signed up to work at the Alcoholic Treatment program in Dix Hall where I would be the group therapist, and at Whiting Forensic Institute I began to serve both in a spiritual and a therapeutic role. Back in New Britain I continued to serve as a pastor.

In Whiting, the population of patients were mostly inmates of the state prison system who were suffering from emotional disturbances. When I did religious services for them I was able to find materials that were both inspirational as well as comforting. I drew upon easily comprehensible quotes from the books of many religions, although my primary source for this group was still one of the dozen or so translations of Christian Bibles which I had collected. My services were attended by Catholics, Protestants...even Black Muslims. When the group was mostly black I learned how to add "call and response" to my homiletic repertoire.

It was also at Whiting that I learned about forensic psychology, psychometrics (psychological testing), and how to work with a population of predominately manipulative, criminal-type personalities. I became increasingly more adept at "smelling a con-job" when I was on the receiving end of one and was the only counselor to correctly diagnose one patient as totally psychopathic when the medical staff saw him as schizophrenic. He had learned how to "play" a schizophrenic. The staff voted to have him returned to court with a recommendation for a verdict of "not guilty by reason of insanity." I opposed this decision but lost. He was judged insane and sent to a full-time psychiatric facility from which he escaped and fled south to be rearrested on abduction and rape charges.

When my training year ran out, I stayed on at Whiting for another six months as a staff counselor. During this time I indicated to my congregation in New Britain that I wanted to become a full-time pastoral counselor and began educating one of its members to take over as the interim pastor until the congregation secured another. This was met with both support and disappointment. As Mr. Bristol took over more and more of the pastoral duties, however, the group was ready to let go. I had a grand farewell party and Sharon and I moved to Bethel to find a job in Western Connecticut on a lead that some friends had given us.

After a four-month search I obtained a position as assistant coordinator of the Day Treatment Program of the Mental Health Clinic of Danbury Hospital. Dr. Richmond Hubbard, the acting director, knew that I was a pastoral counselor, but he was impressed with my knowledge of psychotherapy and gave me the position. I liked him immediately and was pleased with his apparent concern for the patients in day treatment. I was thrilled to have the experience of this job, but my first days at the program were a bit shaky for me. I wanted to go slowly with my new position of leadership in a strictly psychotherapeutic (not spiritual) service function. The shift was not impossible, but it felt difficult. I started out as a group leader, but when the Coordinator quit her position two weeks later, I found the burden of the entire program on my shoulders. I had no staff and over twenty chronically ill, schizophrenic patients to attend to. It was time for me to do a lot more reading and to go back to school. I enrolled at Western Connecticut State College and matriculated in the master's program with a concentration in psychology this time. This wasn't all I did, however.

When I had moved to Bethel, I decided that I should apply for ordination in Unitarian Universalism. It was a religion most similar to my own. I sent all of the application materials to their headquarters in Boston. In anticipation that I would be accepted, I began telling new people that I met that I was a "Unitarian" minister. It was a whole lot simpler than explaining my complicated spiritual background, belief system and training. Years later this "deception" would come back to haunt me. I was never ordained by the U.U.A. and eventually I left the ministry altogether (resigned from the Life Science Church) in favor of psychology. Once I had said that I was a Unitarian minister, however, people knew of me in that capacity, and I was forced to sustain a lie. Many tangled webs proceeded. Maybe this was responsible in some way for the accident? It had to be! I had taken my well-intended spiritual calling and destroyed it with a lie. I believed that I had ascertained the answer to my existential question.

In another week it would be August. I was starting to feel a bit relieved once I had found a reason or purpose for my present suffering. It was a great deal like the "search for meaning" that Victor Frankel describes in his book about his captivity as a Jew in a Nazi death camp. He had even developed a whole form of therapy based upon this existential orientation to problems. He called it Logotherapy. So, using his thinking, I was being punished or, more psychologically, perhaps, I had punished myself for the lies I told about being a Unitarian minister. It seemed plausible. I didn't yet know how close to true guilt I had come.

Maureen, the usual day nurse assigned to me, appeared at my doorway carrying my breakfast tray. She was a very attractive, bright, and friendly individual. I had come to especially appreciate the way she could stay with me, even rest her hand on my shoulder when I cried so heavily. The day nursing staff at White Plains were, in general, excellent "healers."

"Hi, Maureen. You're looking cheerful this morning." Then I wondered if that was a projection of my own happier feelings.

"Yeah. My sister from Denver came to visit us over the weekend and we had a really wonderful time." Maureen was smiling broadly and moving about animatedly as she spoke.

"Hey," I thought to myself with some embarrassment, "I'm getting turned on!" She interrupted my thought.

"I haven't seen her in years and I really had a good time with her again."

"That's great. I can understand the experience of getting together with someone you haven't seen in a long time. I've been doing this a lot lately in the hospital. Are you the eldest of your siblings?"

"No. She's my 'big sister'—eight years older—I really used to love to talk to her about my dating problems when I was growing up."

"That's a coincidence. I have a brother who is ten years older and I used to confide in him quite a bit when I was in school. He was one of my best friends…and sort of like a teacher to me too."

"No kidding?" Maureen looked up momentarily and gave me a wide, toothy smile. "O.K." She then focused her eyes on my face. "Hey, you look much brighter today yourself. Are you accepting things more?"

"I'm not sure," I said looking at her bending forward to place the tray on my bed stand. "I think that I have made some sort of peace with myself this past week and I'm beginning to accept that it happened, not the loss yet. Um…can I ask you a question?"

"Sure." She was now adjusting the thick, plastic pillow that was jammed into the foot of the bed, her back slightly turned toward me. I couldn't keep my eyes off of the round curve of her rear-end, the way the panty line was visible through the white Dacron fabric of her nurse's uniform.

"Well...um...I was wondering. I have been looking down at my legs, or what's left of them, for about two months now. I think that I look ugly. I used to be quite handsome—I even did some modeling for artists as a part-time job—so I was wondering if you thought that anyone would still think that I was good-looking anymore." My voice was trembling. I expected that she would say that I was repulsive.

"Do you want an honest answer?"

"Yes," I said. "No," I thought.

"I think you are very handsome. If I met you someplace outside of this hospital I would think that you were very attractive. I do think that you should shave each day, however."

"Thank you...thank you for what you said." My hand went self-consciously to my face to feel the stubble that was there from several days of not shaving. "I do believe I'll shave today. When I'm finished with breakfast, would you bring me a mirror and razor?"

"No problem." Maureen turned and walked gracefully out of the room. I enjoyed watching her rear-end leave.

After washing and shaving (I hadn't really given the meal much of the usual attention) I rang for a nurse to remove the basin. Pat came in. She was another nurse whom I had grown to appreciate and hold in high regard. Today I didn't see her as my nurse, however. I saw a tall, dark-haired, attractive woman with a great body. What the heck was going on with me? "Oh well...go with the flow," I thought.

When she had gone from the room I eased myself down in the bed and thought about my unusual reaction to those two nurses. I was very aroused. For the first time in months I actually felt undepressed enough to be sexually stimulated. The thought amused me. I let myself drift in and out of sexual reveries for most of the rest of that day. I imagined myself making love to my nurses: one at a time, together, with Carolyn—every combination. It was wonderful to fantasize again. I managed to pull myself away from these pleasant thoughts in the evening when the dinner tray arrived and again when I had two visitors and watched several hours of television. By 10:30 p.m., however, as I began to prepare for sleep, the pleasant sexual fantasies returned. How nice. I decided to masturbate. I rolled over to the right and pulled out the drawer of the nightstand next to the bed. In the single drawer I pushed around the box of Kleenex, several pens, my wristwatch, two *Time Magazines*, a half-eaten bar of Nestle's Crunch and the Keri Lotion. Keri Lotion is the old standby in most hospitals for such things as back rubs, but I had a different use in mind.

The muscles in my belly relaxed as I settled into the slow, building pleasure of masturbating to one of the day's fantasies. I was enjoying the feeling of being undepressed, of feeling sexual again. Several times I stopped just to enjoy the pleasure a bit longer. It had been such a long time. Finally and powerfully the moment of inevitability arrived. My hips lunged forward as I thrust in and out of my hand. Immediately and agonizingly the thought arrived in the very moment following orgasm. "This was the sin of which I was guilty! I had been punished for all of the times I had masturbated in my life!" The guilt descended on me like a hellish weight. My mind reeled with the guilt, with the rising panic. A cold sweat broke out on my forehead as I dropped my head back onto the pillow, the thoughts racing on like a steam engine, the panic building like a different kind of masturbation—one from which there is no release!

This was incomprehensible. I no longer believed in such things. Sure, I had confessed masturbating to a priest every week for fourteen or fifteen years. Yes, I had even cried in the confessional asking forgiveness for something which my body said was natural but the Church said would "cast you into the flames of Hell for all eternity." But I had recovered from this kind of thinking. I had even studied liberal theology!

"I don't believe that masturbation is a sin anymore," my rational mind screamed into the dark, flame-filled void in my brain. This was crazy. Could a childhood, long worked through, long forgotten, have this kind of hold on me? After letting the panic rise to a pitch that made me want to run from the prison of my bed I realized that I had to get some kind of professional assistance with this one. I fumbled for the white tube at the side of the bed with the red button on it. I pressed the button. In a few moments an older, kindly-looking nurse entered the room. I needed to talk to a psychologist.

"Excuse me...but...is there a psychologist on staff on call at this hour?"

"No. But you can have an appointment with one within the next few days if you like."

"I don't know...um...I'm experiencing a great deal of panic right now...uh...I'm not sure how to talk about this with you but I've got to talk to someone right now, please."

"Sure," she said matter-of-factly. "What do you think is making you feel so anxious right now?" That sounded good. She responded to me like a therapist. I felt some trust in her.

"Can I talk to you about anything...uh...something sexual that's bothering me?"

"Certainly. I am a nurse and I have heard a lot of things that were sexual in nature. I also did psych-nursing for a while. So what's bothering you?" I felt safe to take the next risk.

"Well…I was born and raised a Roman Catholic."

She nodded and said, "Uh huh."

"…so anyway, I used to feel very guilty as a child about a lot of things that were sexual. Even sexual thoughts used to make me feel guilty. It was how I was raised. Do you understand what I mean?" She nodded benevolently. "Well…um…I can talk about anything, right?"

"I told you that I am a nurse. I'm a professional. Go on."

"Tonight I masturbated." I looked at her face for a sign of negative reaction. There was none so I went on with some confidence. "I haven't experienced any sexual or joyful feelings in months. I thought it would feel all right, but I immediately felt guilty. I felt like I was a kid again and I can't seem to shake the feeling that I've done something wrong. You can see that I'm sweating right now. I feel hot all over."

"Hot. Like in hell?" she interpreted. I didn't mind. I felt her professionalism coming through and it was comforting.

"Yes…like the reason that I lost my leg had to do with my being sexual. God, I feel guilty right now as I say that to you." You might find what she said next to be absolutely unbelievable, but I swear that it is true.

"You *should feel guilty*! Masturbation *is a mortal sin*, you know! Would you like me to get a priest to hear your confession tomorrow?"

What happened after that I don't remember. I was left in the dark night of my soul. She left somehow. I don't remember what I said to her or how she left. I lay in the dark room with knots in my stomach and a full-blown anxiety attack going on. I was beginning to have trouble breathing. By 3:00 a.m. I had managed to get enough hold of my mind to call upon the therapist within me, the guy with all of the professional training. I decided to facilitate myself in a kind of "two chair," a technique like the one I had used with Albert, getting him to play his mother. The character in the other place would be "God," however.

Me as John: "God…I need you right now. I need your help. Please tell me. Did you take my leg away for some reason?"

Me as God: "No John, I don't do things like that. That is some old-fashioned view of me. I am here to help you in your suffering. I didn't take your leg for any reason. It just happened to you. It was an accident."

John (with tears streaming down my cheeks): "You didn't punish me for anything?" I was still uncertain that I could believe this answer from another part of my psyche.

God: "No. I told you. I'm not that kind of God."

John: "What about my masturbating? Is it a sin?"

God: "Masturbating is sex, right?"

John: "Yes."

God: "Well…I invented sex. I gave it to you to enjoy. There is nothing wrong with your pleasuring yourself."

I felt a shift within me at these last words, or rather, thoughts in my mind. I *knew* that this *was* true. The Catholic child in me who was so uncertain and frightened up until this time was appeased and finally let go. I ended my self-therapy session at around 4:00 a.m. by masturbating again and then falling peacefully to sleep.

CHAPTER 6

The rehabilitation ward at Danbury Hospital was busy that morning. I was one of two new patients who were being admitted and there was so much paperwork to complete, room assignments to make and the usual patients to attend to or monitor. Nurses were scurrying all over the place that day. One patient in Room 14 needed to be specially monitored. He was severely brain damaged from an automobile accident. He probably wouldn't be improving, I later learned, but it was apparently important for the staff to occasionally watch the closed-circuit television in the nurses' station to see what he was up to. I overheard that he had already pulled out his IV several times and they had been forced to permanently restrain him by using soft cuffs fastened at the wrists. These would be connected to the side rails on the bed and would prevent him from grabbing at anything with his hands. He could still aspirate his own saliva, however, and they had to watch him from time to time to see how he was doing. The man in 08 had a severe decubitus. He spent a lot of time at home sitting. He was a paraplegic and had given up trying to get out of the house. He came in on a regular basis. This was the third time this year. He would need routine dressing changes and exposure to a special lamp today. The lamp would kill the staph infection festering in the open ulcer on the bone near the end of his spine. The woman in 11 was in better physical condition, but she was in terrible psychological shape. Only seventeen years old, she had been swimming with friends at Squantz Pond when several of them encouraged her to dive off of the boat dock. She struck her head on a large rock under the water's surface and immediately broke her neck at C-5. She was experiencing the shock of waking up a total quadriplegic, unable to move any part of her body from the neck down. She was psychotically depressed—totally unresponsive—and had to be fed intravenously.

They put me, the return from White Plains Hospital, in room 12. Since I was just "an amputee," I would be there for routine physical and occupational therapy, being fitted with a prosthesis and be discharged at the appropriate time to continue my interrupted life. I was not what you call a very serious case for the unit. My file had arrived with me, but there were some minor irregularities. There was no copy of my medication orders. They would have to wait and see what my physician at Danbury would order for me the next day. That first day they would just give me my meals and help me to settle in. I didn't know at first about my medications.

I was excited. I was back at Danbury Hospital and except for the continuing grief reaction I would have to experience on and off for the next year or two, I was actually feeling quite positive about getting the cast cut off of my amputated leg and getting a prosthesis. My right foot was still in a Hoffman frame but I would be getting that off in the next couple of weeks and learning how to walk again.

Just before lunch time my nurse came in and introduced herself to me. Her name was Ellie and would be assigned to me during the day shift. She had previously been a psychiatric nurse but had worked on the rehab unit for several years now. I immediately liked her. She was genuinely warm and sincere. She seemed to care without being phony-sweet.

We talked for fifteen minutes or so and then she went out to tend to her other patients. In another half hour she brought in my lunch tray. There was no little white paper cup with my noon medications in it. No Haldol. No Dilaudid. No Elavil. No *nothing*!

I didn't think much of it. I hadn't had the morning meds either but maybe they were just cutting down on my dose or they had changed the times when I was to get them. It didn't matter. I was happy to be back in Danbury and on the road to recovery.

The afternoon went well. I read several magazines that I purchased from the bright pink cart which the volunteer had pushed into my room at around 2:30 p.m. She was very helpful in finding an issue of *Popular Photography* for me. I also had bought a candy bar from the cart. It was not a very good grade of chocolate, but it was sweet and satisfied my desire for something other that the usual hospital fare. I began to feel a bit edgy by supper. I couldn't really describe the feeling to anyone. It was kind of like being given five cups of coffee and whacked all over with a hammer. All my joints began to ache. The pain in my right ankle was considerable and my graft donor sites were beginning to burn. There was no cup of medications with supper either. I complained to the nurse but she only said that there "were no orders for meds." I asked her to get in touch with my doctor and "get some orders for pain killers." She said she'd try. By 8:00 p.m., the pain was horrible but no one had been able to get a physician's instructions to administer any medications. By 10:00 p.m. the restlessness had increased markedly. I gripped the bed rails and bit down on my pillow to fight the pain and the nervous feelings. I wanted to get out of the bed. I felt obsessed with the desire to run…to scream…to walk down to the nurses' station and demand a medication. I pushed the button again.

Ruth came almost immediately.

"Hasn't anyone been able to contact Foster yet? I'm feeling really lousy right now. The pain is more than I've felt in a long time and I also feel like I've got to get out of the bed. I think the restlessness is from not having any tranquilizer…you know, Ruth?"

"I know, John…but there's nothing we in the nursing staff can do right now without a doctor's orders. We can't give you anything…except…" She bent her head in thought for a moment. "Well, we can give you Tylenol?"

"Oh boy, Ruth. You know as well as I do that Tylenol is not going to do the trick, not after being on a major tranquilizer and a morphine derivative for the past two months."

"I know, John. I really wish that there was something I could do. It's a real foul up, but we're stuck here too." She looked so concerned about wanting to help me in view of the mess up in orders.

"O.K., Ruth, all right. I'll take the Tylenol. But please see if you can get a hold of Foster or anybody—an intern or resident—if you have to. I have to get back on those medications. I'm clearly physically dependent now."

"I'll do the best I can." I knew that this was the truth.

The Tylenol didn't anesthetize anything. It might as well have been another cup of coffee for how I was feeling by midnight. On top of this, there was one female patient on the ward that kept calling out, "Harold. Harold…oh help me Harold. Please, in the name of Jesus Christ, our Lord and Savior…merciful Jesus…Harold! I'm your mother. Oh God in heaven, almighty…Harold!!" I began to feel sorry for the poor lady but also I started to feel like I was now in a psych ward instead of rehab.

I decided to do pull-ups on the trapeze apparatus above the bed. I figured the exercise might wear me out and take my mind off of my pain…and the woman. I exercised until I couldn't pull myself up any more. My arms were just too tired but the restless feeling, not to mention the delirious woman, was positively maddening. After a brief rest I actually succeeded in getting myself partially out of the bed and seated in the yellow arm chair on the left. My foot ached from the new direction of pull created by my change in body position relative to the weights of the traction device, but I just had to get out of bed, even if only a few feet! The night nurse caught me.

"What are you doing?" She sounded quite agitated.

"...Harold!! Oh God, Jesus Christ...I died for your sins, Harold..."

"I'm trying to feel better!" I was angry, frustrated.

"If you don't get back in that bed right now I will get someone to restrain you to the bed. Do you understand?"

"...kill me. They want to..."

"What?" The word "restrain" scared me. Immediately I had visions of being tied up like a mental patient in one of the state hospitals I had worked in during my early training in therapy. Those were not pretty memories. I obeyed.

"Now. What exactly is going on here?" She was stern.

"...Oh Heavenly Father...in Heaven...Jesus, Mary and Joseph..."

"Look. I haven't had any Dilaudid or any of my other medications all day. I feel like shit. My joints are aching too and I think I'm going into withdrawal."

"Don't get excited. I'll try to get in touch with your doctor and see what we can get for you. I'm sorry if I sounded too threatening before, but you worried me."

"HAROLD!!!"

"That's O.K." I began to feel a little hope. "Just do what you can. Oh...and could you please close the door to the room of the lady down the hall?"

"Sure." Within another minute, the woman's voice took on a muffled, background quality. I shed a few tears for her and then settled down into my pain and agitation. I would wait for my doctor.

By 3:00 a.m. I could barely push the red button. My hands were shaking considerably. I was sweating profusely and was having violent, involuntary contractions of most of the muscles in my body. I felt scared, agitated and I was in a tremendous amount of physical pain. Pain comes in all varieties. I was having them all: dull aches in the joints, sharp, lancing, and throbbing pains in the graft donor sites on my right thigh, pulling pains in my right foot, "phantom" crushing pains in my missing leg, strong aches in the ankle bones of the real foot and stinging pains at the pin sites in my right shin. My mind was alternately racing and slumping into a kind of incoherence. I felt her presence through a fog.

"I'm in withdrawal," I mumbled through parched lips. I was sweating so much but my throat was dry. "Help me. Please."

"There's nothing we can do. No one ever dies from going 'cold turkey.'

You *are* having a withdrawal reaction now and that makes sense considering what you told the last nurse about the kinds of medications you were on, but there's nothing we can do until your doctor comes in tomorrow." She was holding onto my left arm just above the wrist. I imagined that she was trying to do what little she could under the circumstances to ameliorate my unpleasant state of affairs but my body was doing what it was doing *without* my voluntary or emotional control. There was no way she could calm it or me down. I was convulsing by sunrise and began to come down before 7:00 a.m. By 10:00 I was looking at the tall, white, lab coat once more.

"You have no idea what I've been through during the night," I said with a sarcastic tone in my voice.

"I heard that you had drug withdrawal. I'm really sorry about that, John. I've written orders for most of your medications—I'm taking you off Haldol—and a nurse will be in shortly with your Dilaudid. How are you feeling right now?" His voice was soft and soothing.

"I hurt a lot but most of the restless, jumpy feeling is gone. I've watched other people in detox units go through withdrawal from heroin or alcohol but I'd never have imagined that someday I would experience it first-hand. It was really weird."

"You are a tough guy, John, to have gone through all that you've been through so far...and then to have to suffer this indignity as well." He was shaking his head sympathetically. "I'm sorry."

I believed him. Craig Foster was and is one of the most dedicated physicians I've ever met. I would have—and have—trusted him with my life. I felt satisfied. Moments later Ellie was giving me a shot of analgesic medication, and I felt my body relaxing and slipping into the soft, dull ache with which I was more familiar.

By the end of July I was getting fairly eager to get on with the rehabilitation program designed for my particular injuries. I had come back to Danbury Hospital to get rehabilitated—to actively participate in the programs that would lead to becoming more independent—and nothing had happened for the prior four days. I was still flat on my back, waiting and waiting and waiting. I wished at times that I were the kind of person who could sit around all day, get tired reading or writing and then sleep soundly at night—I didn't know how paraplegics did it—but I knew that I needed to be much more physically active somehow. Even a whole day of visitors or exercise with arm weights didn't allow me to sleep well at night. It really came down to needing more total mobility. As I had noted in White Plains, the healing process had increased my body energy markedly. In addition, Craig had taken me off of a major tranquilizer, and that tended to give me a more natural disposition to want to get out of bed.

I began to develop a daily regimen of pull ups on the trapeze apparatus above the bed. I thought, "I still feel full of vigor, full of life, ready to go. While my arms are tired, the exercise does nothing to tire me at all. This feeling is what one must call 'chomping at the bit.' Just turn me loose in the P.T. room and I'll get the rehabilitation that I need to get out of here, and I'll also sleep better at night."

On July 29th I had been visited by friends from the Unitarian Universalist Society of which I was a member. One of the things that was so memorable about this visit was that Darius brought in a felt dart board and we threw velcro-covered balls at it for a while. It helped to relieve a great deal of the boredom. I loved it. I found it easy to be interested in what we were doing. How nice for a change.

Within the next three days I expected to see Foster at 11:00 a.m. but a half hour before his expected arrival he called to say that he would have to change that to 6:00 p.m. "Another 8 hours of waiting!" I lamented. Even after all of my years of sedentary work as a psychotherapist, patiently watching the process of other people while sitting, almost motionless in a chair, I had not prepared myself for the incredible patience required of a four-month hospital stay. When Foster arrived, I decided I would say nothing to him about the long wait, I merely would request a wheelchair order. On a previous occasion, he had said he would give it the "utmost consideration provided that my right leg could withstand being lowered below the level of my heart [increased blood pressure in the arteries of the foot] and that my brain could handle the orthostatic hypotension [sudden drop in blood pressure in the brain as the blood rushed into the legs]." I had nodded in understanding.

To pass the time I once again tried to think of things to occupy time. The previous day, Vinny, another patient who appeared to have some kind of brain damage affecting the expressive areas of his brain and some of his motor functions, brought me a newspaper so I could have something to read. I felt really touched by this. That was really kind of him. I was unable to have much of a meaningful conversation with him, but I tried to express my gratitude clearly. His appearance reminded me that I might also be ready for some distracting, intellectual stimulation. "This hospitalization thing is just so fucking boring. I wonder how anyone (most people hate to stay in bed with so much as a cold) could lie so patiently, be in one position for three months...or in a Striker frame. Wow...what a horrible concept!" I thought. I rolled over and looked out the window at the grey sky over Danbury. "God...I wish they'd do some medical procedure on me today," I thought as I rolled over onto my back once again and stared at the ceiling. As if my prayers had been answered I heard a knock at the door.

X-ray came in and did a couple of shots of my ankle. I always liked the procedure because it kept me quite occupied and interested. I watched as they rolled the portable X-ray machine over to the bed, took down the side rails and swung the "head" of the apparatus over my right tibia and fibula. There was a great deal of adjustment to be made, and I enjoyed watching the lead-aproned technicians as they measured distances, placed the photographic plate gently beneath my leg and eventually took the picture. They repeated the process several times, and after about a 40-minute diversion, they left. At 3:00 I thought, "X-ray is gone, all procedures are finished for now and I've got three more hours until Foster arrives. Waiting!...What a pain to be...W...A...I...T...I...N...G." I stretched out the word in my mind as I stared at the perfect, unbroken, cobweb-free, unstreaked ceiling.

"Didn't come at six," I noticed as dinner ended and I glanced at my watch. I felt irritated but got control of my feelings. He probably had a billion things to do to keep his day fulfilling. At 7:00 p.m. he arrived.

The familiar, tall, white lab coat swept into the door and Craig flowed over to the side of the bed. "It's odd how graceful this big guy is," I thought.

"I'm really sorry I'm late, but I had several calls from the emergency room today and I've been really busy."

"Oh...that's O.K.," I lied as nonchalantly as possible.

Anticipating my question, he said, "How'd you like to get out of this bed tomorrow?"

"You're kidding! Would I? I would be ecstatic!" I pushed my way up onto my pillows to look him straight in the face to see if he was just giving me a rhetorical question. He appeared serious. Then he smiled.

Through his obvious happiness he said, "I'll go write the orders for it right now. You'll have to take it carefully due to the changes in blood pressure as I told you before."

I nodded my understanding.

"...but you can spend at least an hour or two in the chair depending on how you feel. I'll also be changing the cast on the stump, but I think it's really too soon to consider the Hoffman apparatus. It has got to be on a bit longer to assure that the bones are knitting properly."

He looked pleased at my reaction to his news. He wished me a comfortable day, and headed for the door. As an afterthought, he pivoted back toward me and advised in a voice a mother might use with her teenage son who is about to borrow the family car for the first time, "Take it easy the first day. I know you've waited a long time for this. Don't overdo it, O.K.?"

"No problem, Craig. Thank *you* very much," I said. "Thank God," I thought to myself.

The next day I was taught how to transfer, using a special board, from the side of the bed to the wheelchair. I had no difficulty with the transfer. My arms were quite strong and I lifted myself up with ease. I was delighted to be up after so many days of waiting and lying in bed, but I was also quite surprised that the ward was not larger. "There's really not much to it...except maybe the lounge. So far I only see a larger T.V. in there," I thought. A bigger television was not what I needed. Physical therapy was.

I liked working out on the weights at the wall...with the pulleys. My arms actually ached (that good kind of hurt) and I literally began to feel tired after a good long workout. Every day I got stronger and stronger. I still made unfortunate comparisons between my new life and the former one. I remembered myself doing ballet and jazz dancing, modeling, and walking barefoot in the sand. "I'll never feel the sand or grass on my bare feet again," was one realization.

In early August Foster did another procedure. He put a new cast on my stump, removed the dressing from my right thigh and found infections of the graft sites. The plastic Opcite had to be removed. It was like having strapping tape pulled off of a burn. The procedure hurt like hell. I thought I was going to pass out at one point. The Metz's, friends from Arizona, held my hand while I cried out and then a nurse brought me some chocolate ice cream which I devoured gratefully. I felt like a kid who had just gotten a lollypop at the dentist's office. Strange, how this "goody" worked with me as an adult—well maybe as a regressed adult anyway. I spent a precious hour in my wheelchair later that evening.

Some of the improvements that accompanied moving to a wheelchair were being able to wear a T-shirt in place of a "Johnny coat" and getting special shorts from Carolyn that were split up the sides with velcro sewn on for closure. I put the shorts on by passing them between my crotch and then fastening them at the sides. They worked very well and I felt infinitely more civil wearing them.

Off and on over the next week I found myself crying. I regarded it as a healthy part of the overall grief process and welcomed the relief that came from letting these feelings out. I no longer had any repression about my feelings, and my depression was quite under control by early August.

I could see that I was ready to get back to work on my doctoral program again and even wished I could begin seeing clients. I fantasized about having a room in the rehab unit where I would be doing therapy or doing something of value and service. This, of course, would never come to be, but I could always get back to studying for my oral boards in my doctoral program.

Finally, when Carolyn was visiting, I asked her to get for me a whole list of text books for my graduate work and the preliminary study notebooks from my dissertation research. Frankly, I felt quite insecure about getting back into this stuff, but my mind was clear enough to do it, so I said, "...here goes." After Carolyn left, a new nurse came in to tend to me. Her name was "Gagnon." I seldom met Gagnons and was curious about her family's background. She said that her family name (actually the husband's) was, like mine, French Canadian. I gave her Ernie's name, address and telephone number for a genealogy of our line of Gagnon. I hoped that it would be of some use to her husband in figuring out their own family tree. After she left I had several very friendly visitors and a few phone calls.

One of the most striking visits was from another member of our Unitarian universalist Society who worked with plants. Ursula brought me some flowers, herbs, and an entire tree. Someone had told her that I loved the smell of the juniper tree and she brought one that was five feet tall into my room. While the herbs and flowers in their respective pots were nice to look at, the juniper tree filled the room with a wonderful outdoor fragrance. If I closed my eyes I could imagine being in a decidious forest on a cool, summer night. It was a lovely thought.

Carolyn and Isabelle then returned and brought all of the books and papers I requested. I was grateful for the chance to begin my work, but when I saw my family together I felt so damned homesick. "Oh, man, but I miss you guys and I want to be home with you again," I said. There were no dry eyes in the room. I would really have liked to just hug Carolyn again for a very long while (an hour might do). I missed the cottage as well. I wondered how the summer had been on the lake that year. Carolyn told me that she planted lots of flowers all around the stone-marked areas on either side of the front door. I looked forward to seeing that.

My doctoral dissertation involved doing therapy with musicians. I had a great deal of reading to do on the work that had already been done in several fields of music and psychological application. The search of the literature which I did from the hospital room went well. I wrote and rewrote at least three dozen pages of my dissertation while I was there. It occupied my mind in a number of ways and even helped to reduce the pain that came from the infected graft sites and the crushed ankle. This latter item was of no small concern since the rate at which the ankle healed would determine when the Hoffman would come off—that is, when I would learn to walk again. Part of the problem was the continuous bleeding from the foot. As I sat in bed I could often smell my ankle and thigh bandages full of blood and serious discharge. It was a rather strange experience but it was an olfactory measure of progress. As the smell decreased I knew that the areas were healing.

The next time that Carolyn visited she stayed for almost two hours. It was a good visit that gave me a break from my studying and writing. "She's looking tired," I realized. I wished she could have stayed there longer and just lay down and fallen asleep next to me, but she wanted to leave to pick up Isabelle. She was very, very responsible throughout my entire hospitalization. Sometimes it was very stressful for her to be this way and I often checked with friends to make certain that she was being taken care of in some way.

By mid August I was starting to do what is designated "weight bearing" on the right foot. I was placed on a device called a "tilt table". This medieval contraption was a slab of steel that had a supportive plate at one end against which one could rest a real or artificial foot. The angle of the device determined the percentage of body weight that would be transferred to the supporting extremity. My first day on the machine I could take a tilt-table angle of 20 degrees. That felt like a major success in spite of the amount of bleeding I did. Before I was off of the table, the suture lines had all split open, and I had left a fairly sizeable puddle on the floor. I remembered when I hurt my ankle from a Judo throw in high school and how long it took to get back the ability to bend it and put my weight on it. I realized that the present injury would probably take a much longer time. It was my goal to increase the angle of the tilt table a bit more each day.

The next day I increased the angle to 30 degrees and, in spite of more bleeding, felt satisfied by the progress. Later I told Carolyn about the headway. Ted Peatte came in while she was still there, and he recounted the details of my accident to me. It was both fascinating and a little disconcerting to listen to him describe some of those things. Up until that moment I still had not dreamed at night about anything. I still believed that the medication was most likely responsible for preventing dreaming. A funny coincidence, however, happened that day. After Carolyn and Ted left I started to doze off and I felt like I was in some kind of dark place. Everything seemed so dark—like a pitch-black void. I thought I heard a voice say, "He's shocky as hell....He's still alive though..."—something like that. I wondered if that was what a flashback was all about or if this was my first dream.

In physical therapy they began to get me to do leg exercises along with the triceps and biceps curls. I started with quadriceps extensions. Over the months of inactivity the muscles in my legs had atrophied and even if the tilt table could have gotten me up to 90 degrees, it is unlikely that I would have had the strength at this time to stand on my own.

When Carolyn stopped by before she went to work in the nursery, she looked unusually tired and overworked. I felt really sorry for her. I told all of my visitors that week that what I really wanted from them was to take care of Carolyn. I hoped that they would do that, and I checked on their involvement from time to time. I don't know if Carolyn knew I was looking out for her, but one day she gave me a get-well card that said, "You Are My NIGHT LIGHT." It felt good to be taking care of her from the hospital. I also had her withdraw some of my savings to pay bills. I would not let her be burdened by finances without my continuing assistance.

On August 15th, a Wednesday, Stacey David taught me a blessing for the Sabbath: "Baroch utu Adonoi elohainu melech ha uhlum a sher kee-reeshanu bamitz e foesuv vits eevahnu lehadleek nere shell shabot." She spent the whole afternoon with me talking about the research project with musicians. It was delightful. She also gave me a tape of flute music with my favorite piece on it. She had actually found the ensemble for cello, flute and piano by Martinu. Whenever I played it I felt like I was back at Sue Casa, at the first of my musicians' workshops. I also felt anxious to go back to doing the research with musicians for my dissertation. After Stacey left, I decided to call Larry Huntley, head of the music department at Western Connecticut State University, to see about a second year's research group for the fall.

CHAPTER 7

In 1976, I had completed my master's degree in psychology. I was the first graduate from Western Connecticut State College with a major in psychology. The M.S. was an important step for me educationally. It opened up a wider range of other educational opportunities. I could then go to postgraduate institutions such as Ridgelea Institute and the Gestalt Institute of Connecticut. Here I could learn about Gestalt therapy, a form of psychotherapy which allows the therapist to be much more active in his work, facilitating various experiments for the client to experience directly. In this way a client learns how to build his *own* support and be less dependent on the therapist.

I found this Gestalt therapy to be positively exciting. It seemed to approach with clarity and practical vitality client issues I considered to be over-analyzed by the psychodynamic schools or overcontrolled by the behavioral schools. I didn't realize how effective it was, however, until several months after my father died in January of 1976.

I was still working at the Day Treatment Program, now called the Day Hospital and I, then Director, had acquired or been given additional staff. I had secured an occupational therapist, a social worker, an art therapist, a medicating psychiatrist, a dance therapist, a sculpting teacher, and a poetry therapist. My supervisor asked me to write a grant proposal to be submitted to the State of Connecticut. While I was never given credit for the proposal, we were awarded the grant of $50,000. I then interviewed and hired a full-time psychologist and full-time occupational therapist.

There were also more funds for materials and supplies for the various therapies used in the program.

Things had been going well at work, but my mood was greatly affected during the time my father was dying of cancer. I began to get very concerned about how depressed I was feeling and about keeping up the quality of my work in spite of my feelings. Besides administrative duties, I ran groups, saw some patients on an individual basis, administered biofeedback as required for stress, kept up with the paperwork, handled all of the interfaces between the program and the outside psychiatric community, and otherwise dealt with the mental health clinic and the hospital that employed me. My depression contained a great deal of denial about my father. Something seriously needed to be finished with my father, but I didn't know what that was. Whenever I visited home we had, at Mom's demand, denied that he was dying. This was a huge mistake. Neither he nor I ever got a chance to say goodbye or to talk about the years of mutual alienation. I needed to get some psychotherapy myself.

From October of 1975 until June of 1976 I went into therapy with a classical analyst. He nodded patiently as I talked, with free-association, about almost anything. I never felt connected to him or to the therapy, and my depression progressively got worse. My marriage was also greatly affected. Sharon and I were arguing frequently and we had even begun to discuss divorce or maybe an "open marriage." She was being approached sexually by one of the physicians at Danbury Hospital where she worked on the orthopedics ward, and I was interested in a woman colleague. Everything seemed precarious in my life, and the analytic therapy was not helping at all. It was in July of 1976, feeling suicidally depressed, that I decided to go to a Gestalt therapist that several of my friends had recommended to me. His name was George Anderheggen.

I called, made the appointment and came, grey-faced, bags under my eyes, to his office. While my former therapist had never remarked on how I looked or what he sensed about me, George, upon seeing me for the first time said without hesitation, "God...you look like shit!" I immediately burst into tears, crying openly and wrackingly for the first time since I had lain my father in his grave. I leaned forward toward George and he asked if I wanted to be held. I nodded "yes" and he came over to me and embraced me as I sobbed my heart out to him about my father. I talked about the lack of communication that my father and I had throughout his life, of the difficult time we had working together, how he once took me fishing and when I fell in the water, losing his favorite pole, he refused to ever take me fishing again. We accomplished in one session what the analyst couldn't help me to get at in nine months. I was amazed. Within only a few weeks I was out of my depression. I was feeling much better at home and in my job. I decided then and there that I had to study Gestalt therapy. I wanted to be a Gestalt therapist.

I approached the Gestalt Institute of Connecticut. After a rigorous interview and application procedure I was accepted, and by the early fall of 1976 I began one year of specialized training in this treatment methodology. I loved Gestalt therapy, an integrated system of all approaches to therapy. It utilizes any possible theoretical base or technique that is necessary for the client during a particular period in the client's therapy. The therapist always maintains an "I-thou" equal relationship with the client and employs many "experiments" to help the person help himself. When certain persons in therapy are holding back on expression of feelings because of the way in which they are contracting various muscle groups in the neck or shoulders, the Gestalt therapist might ask the client to focus all of his attention upon those muscles, causing historical material, verbal recollections as well as feelings, to surface. The results are astonishing to observe. I was amazed at how fast, accurate, and sensitive Gestalt therapy is. When a new school of therapy arises like Rational Emotive Therapy or Kohutian Analysis for Self Disorders, the Gestalt therapist integrates this body of knowledge into his method. The repertoire of approaches available to the Gestalt therapist is limitless and only restricted if the therapist is not fully attuned to himself and to the client in the individual moments of the therapy process. I was impressed and I studied hard.

I took additional workshops with Dr. George Cloutier, a psychiatrist who ran an entire treatment facility for persons diagnosed as chronic schizophrenic. At this clinic in Maine *no* medication was ever used. When I stayed at the community as a guest trainer I never witnessed any sign of psychotic behavior or thinking from the "patients." This had a tremendous influence on what I began to introduce into my work with patients at the Day Hospital. As I carefully and sensitively used Gestalt therapy with my patients I saw remarkable changes in their behavior. Where previously there was only stagnation and impasse in their lives I saw improvement...even, dare I use the word, cure!

Bill was a new patient to the program. He was just twenty years old and had been hospitalized for the first time a year prior for an acute schizophrenic episode following surgery. He had entered the hospital for cancer in the lymph nodes of the axilla (under the right arm) and the surgery required the removal of many nodes and part of the surrounding musculature. As a result, Bill could not move his hand very well and often had to position it with his left hand. Bill had been an art major in college. He was now considerably weakened and showed a great deal of bizarre and erratic behavior. He began to hallucinate actively approximately one week prior to admission to the Day Hospital.

When Bill arrived, he complained of visual hallucinations (among other difficulties). After several weeks of orientation to the program, he agreed to work on these hallucinations in a group therapy session. He had already done some preliminary work in the group and was familiar with seeing other patients do Gestalt therapy.

The session began with Bill describing the hallucinations, which usually occurred at bedtime and just before sleep. He told the staff that he saw "green faces." Hideous and frightening, these images would loom toward him menacingly from the foot of the bed. He became too frightened to sleep and the images would last for hours. After a lengthy description of the images, I instructed Bill to lie on the floor as if in his bed and to visualize the faces in a chair placed opposite him. He not only imagined them, he told us that he clearly saw them and became frightened. I encouraged him to talk to the faces and then to get up and play them in whatever way he wished. Although he was, at first, reluctant to change positions and was not forced to move, he voluntarily did switch positions and became the Faces.

First as Bill: "Go away. Leave me alone!" Bill said, as he began to whimper and shudder. He repeated this several times and then waited out his reluctance to change places and sit in the position of the Faces. With gentle support from me, he got up and moved to the place where the hallucination hung in the air like a specter.

"That's it, Bill," I coaxed. "See if you can play the part of the green faces for us so we can see just what they look like...you just *play* the part. O.K.?"

Nodding his understanding Bill began as the Faces. "Aaaaagh," he said, making the frightening sound deep in the back of his throat. "We are here to get you." The fingers of his left hand began to clench. He pointed the partly closed hand like a claw at the "bed" position.

"Can you use your hand even more, Faces? Be aware of what your hand is doing."

"Aaaaaagh." He lunged forward with his claw as if to tear Bill's face.

"You look like you want to hurt Bill. Do you want to hurt him?" I spoke easily and without any fear of Bill's Faces.

"We want to kill him!"

"You want to *kill* Bill. Come back now and be Bill again." Bill moved back and forth several times between the two positions with the dialogue taking on repeated versions of the same theme: "I want you to leave me alone!" vs. "I want to kill you." Finally, he returned once more to the "Bill" position. This time he seemed to really hear the message from the Faces. He lay on the floor, wide-eyed, and with his body very, very tense.

"O.K. Bill. Would you experience what you are feeling in your body right now." I suspected that Bill had been cutting off these feelings for a long time now and that I had to proceed very carefully.

"Oh no!" Bill's body trembled and his lips began to quiver as if he would soon cry.

"Oh no, what, Bill?"

"They want to *kill* me!" He looked very frightened and began to gurgle a frothy scream in the back of his throat. He stopped momentarily and looked pleadingly at me for help.

"They want to kill you?...I'm here with you right now, Bill, and I think you really look scared. Would you like some help?" I leaned forward on one knee.

"No. No. I'm not frightened!" his eyes became more spacey but his voice raised in pitch and volume, the tone becoming strident.

Going with the need to deny, I encouraged, "O.K.... Tell them that.... Say, 'I'm not frightened of you and I'm not frightened of your killing me.'"

Beginning, "I'm not frightened of you..." Bill suddenly opened his eyes wide again. He began a rising pitched scream. He wrapped his arms around himself as if to keep his body from flying apart.

Moving forward again, I offered, "Would you like to be held right now, Bill? May I hold you?"

Nodding pleadingly, Bill rolled into my arms. I held him the way that Bill had been holding himself. Bill's screaming became deeper and louder. His muscles, which had been chronically rigid for months, began to relax and he began to cry heavily. I experienced his positive reaction to being held and held Bill more tightly. Bill's crying went on for quite a while with him being held tightly throughout. At one point Bill looked up and screamed, "The light!" The room was dimly lit. "The light...it hurts my eyes!" Was this the light that had shown down on his body as it lay on the operating table over one year before?

Bill then began to reach a natural calm and I held him more lightly as I rocked him gently for a long time. Finally, Bill sat up with assistance from Christy, the art therapist, and smiled at the group. He made *clear eye contact* this time! "I was...so...scared. I was afraid of dying. I know I've been afraid of dying for a long time now."

"Do you think you are dying now, Bill?" I asked kindly.

After a thoughtful (feelingful) pause Bill answered, "Nope." He smiled, again with the same strong, clear eye contact.

"O.K., Bill. Do you feel like you could do a bit more now or would you like to stop for today? See how you feel about it."

Bill looked at the floor as he thought, searched his inner self to see if he really wanted to go on. This was not the impulsive behavior of a schizophrenic patient, it was the normal cognitive, self-aware processing of a normal individual. "Sure. I'm tired but I'm O.K. enough to do a bit more." He then indicated to us that he would stop if he wanted (another sign of an internal locus of control). He nodded again to give more impact to his words and again made strong eye contact with me.

"O.K., Bill. Become the Faces again if you would."

Bill got up again and walked confidently to the spot where he had played the Faces before. As he arrived, his face took on a more sinister look.

"What are you feeling right now?" I queried, imagining the answer ahead of time.

"I'm feeling evil and deadly." His voice had a sardonic quality to it.

"You're evil and deadly...but not to Bill anymore?"

"Right! But everyone else better watch out because I'm very evil." Bill laughed as he felt his power turned outward for the first time in a year.

"Be Bill again." He changed positions, somewhat reluctantly this time. "Do you see the Faces, Bill?"

"No. Not any more. I could imagine that I was the Faces but I don't actually see them."

"Such reality testing," I thought quietly to myself.

"I could make believe..."

I felt pleased with Bill's willingness to get into owning more of his angry energy but felt that the session had gone long enough for one day. "O.K., Bill," I laughed. "I know how good that must have felt but let's stop here for now...."

For the next week Bill reported no hallucinations. He was able to speak much more clearly to members of the staff and actually began painting again, teaching himself to use his left hand. His fear had decreased considerably and he was not projecting his anger onto anyone or anything. He expressed how angry he was about his surgery and about the loss of the use of his right hand. Bill decided to work again several sessions later. I asked him if he would be willing to experiment with the Faces again. He was very willing and was able to make the transition between the "Bill" and the "Faces" position with ease. He again actually seemed to enjoy the power of being the angry Faces. This time I asked Bill to try an experiment in which he would go around the group and show the Faces to people in the group. He did this gleefully and felt stronger afterward. It was in this playing out of the frightening and aggressive Faces that Bill made tremendous progress. This was where his integration of the split-off aggression seemed to occur. His whole demeanor changed after this. If anyone has ever seen the face of one mired in the swamp of schizophrenia, one can appreciate the difference in facial expressions that Bill underwent. He became more energetic and confident. He did not have any further hallucinations and seemed much more lucid. The green "surgical mask faces" never appeared again. This was the power and effectiveness of Gestalt therapy in action.

Jane had been a regular patient at the Day Hospital for several months. She suffered mostly from delusions or, more accurately, from one particular delusion of "Sin and Guilt." As she put it, "I believe I'm totally evil for saying swear words in my head." An ex-Catholic, Jane believed that there was no hope for her. She also believed that any priest who saw her would immediatly know that she "was evil" and would never forgive her in confession.

I began her work in one session by suggesting an experiment where she try to change some of the statements she made about guilt into statements of resentment. This came from my learning to appreciate guilt as frequently being retroflected resentment (a negative feeling turned back upon oneself). These resentful expressions were at first difficult for Jane to make but came more easily with repeated experimentation. Most of the statements of resentment came out as directed against the Church. She found that she resented many of the rules which the Church had made about "impure or evil" thoughts. In one session I decided to let Jane "become the Church" to have the power of rule-making and forgiveness. I set up two separate chairs where Jane could be herself in the one place and a "priest in a confessional" in the other. Jane moved freely between her chair and the priest's. She dialogued at length about what things were in fact sinful and what were not. As the priest she began to change some of the rules about swearing and was able to, in her words, "grant Jane absolution for any sins which she might actually have committed" according to a more reasonable ethos. She gave herself a penance of prayers that she could perform in order to get total forgiveness and was delighted at the relief she felt once she began to own the power of forgiving herself.

The entire treatment using repeated confessional scenes lasted eight sessions, at the end of which Jane said, "I can now guiltlessly (though appropriately) swear out loud or in my head." Therapists sometimes swore with her or at one another or other patients as appropriate. When someone acted really self-destructively, a therapist might be heard to say, "You are acting like an asshole, Frank." Therapists were free to insult one another in a similar way when provoked. Jane and a number of other patients learned to accept this as a natural way of expressing disapproval without it being sinful. She no longer felt hopeless and was able to discuss with clarity how destructive certain aspects of her religious background had been to her. Most importantly, she felt like she could now forgive herself for things she might do which violated her own ethics (though she very much wanted to follow the dictates of her conscience). Jane reowned her projected, critical self and even became *less* critical in the process.

In Gestalt therapy, many patients benefited from interventions that accomplished in a few sessions what more than several years in the state hospital had failed to achieve.

Danny, a 15-year-old boy was often withdrawn and fearful, although he could be quite verbal when he wanted. He believed that he was constantly being watched. He never looked at anyone but assumed that people were staring at him critically. Occasionally, he would look up at someone and see that person looking back. Danny would then avert his gaze and persist with the (grandiose) idea that he was being watched. His eyes often appeared glassy and unfocused. His favorite place in the group room was a dark isolated corner.

In one session, after several preliminary attempts to make eye contact with Danny, I was able to coax him to try an experiment.

"Danny, are you aware that you haven't looked at me at all during the session?"

Leaning to one side and shuffling his feet. "Uh…no. Well…I mean…I suppose not."

"You *suppose* not?" I emphasized the words so Danny could hear the indirectness of his own speech.

"Yeah…." He began to fiddle with his fingers. "…uh…I don't like people staring at me." His finger movements became more frantic. "It makes me uncomfortable."

"Do you feel uncomfortable right now?"

"Yeah…I feel like you hate me or something. I don't know." He shifted uneasily back and forth in the chair, his eyes averted downward.

"Would you be willing to try something?"

"What?" Danny looked very suspicious.

I leaned back in my folding chair and place my hands in my lap. "Would you try looking at me and see what I look like?"

Shuffling uncomfortably again, Danny replied, "Yeah, I guess so….Yeah…sure." He raised his eyes and looked glassily for a moment. Then his eyes went wide and he quickly returned his gaze to the worn, brown carpet.

"What did you see, Danny?"

"Nothing much…just you."

"Did I look hateful?" I queried.

"A little." He nodded in agreement with himself.

"Danny, would you try to keep your eyes on me for as long as you can and see me even though I might look hateful to you right now? You can stop whenever you feel too uncomfortable to go on."

He looked up. He nodded slowly. His eyes widened again and he appeared frightened and unfocused.

I nodded at Danny's efforts. "Good. That's it, Danny. See if you can stay with the looking. Do you feel anything right now?"

"Yeah...I feel...scared!"

I then encouraged the frightened young man to experience even more of his fear by becoming "more aware of how the fear feels." Danny first attempted to control the emerging feelings by not shaking and by keeping his breathing shallow. I instructed him to be aware of both of these things and he began to shake more profoundly. After a few moments, Danny started to cry. His crying kept up for about five minutes with shaking and, at times, deep sobbing. After this time, Danny stopped shaking, maintained looking at me and relaxed. His shoulders dropped visibly. His eyes appeared to come into focus.

"What's happening, Danny?" I said in a tender voice.

"I was really scared of you I guess, but I feel better now."

"Let's end for now, Danny, O.K.?" I would finish this work with Danny at another time.

In subsequent sessions Danny was asked to repeat the contact experiment with me and alternately withdraw into himself. He was instructed to say to himself with each behavior, "I can be in contact. I can withdraw." Danny began to learn to appreciate both movements or behaviors. He carried out this exercise with ease after a while. In one session I gave him pleasant scenes from books to focus on for periods of time, after which he made a few moments of eye contact with me. Danny was able to maintain eye contact for longer and longer periods of time without discomfort. Eventually, I offered Danny an experiment that would give him back his visual aggression.

"Danny, would you be willing to make some eye contact with a few members of the group and try to scare them with your eyes?"

"I guess so. I mean....I'll do it...I'll try, anyway." He smiled at his increased sense of assertiveness. He got up tentatively and approached a female group member. He bent forward and looked hatefully at her. Her eyes widened slightly and she fidgeted a bit. Danny stood back looking pleased.

"What happened? What was that like for you?" I asked, already knowing what Danny's answer would be.

"Great! I think I really scared her." His voice was pleased and his cheeks glowed with a little color. This was a nice thing to see in one who usually looked so pale, so lifeless.

"You enjoyed scaring her?"

"Yeah. Now *I* get to be scary for a change."

Later, Danny was able to repeat this experiment with other members of the group, and, although he did not always scare others, he became pleased with the aggressive use of his eyes. He was able to take this experiment outside of the Day Hospital with him and found great comfort and satisfaction in looking aggressively at others. Danny became less withdrawn in the program and participated more and more in the group activities. His fears had decreased significantly through what was, for him, a safer and self-empowering use of his eyes to see what was really there.

I was very pleased with the many positive things I experienced doing Gestalt therapy at the Day Hospital, and I wanted to learn to do more for our patients. I developed an educational consortium with the University of Bridgeport and Western Connecticut State College, social work department. I became a co-founder of the Partial Hospitalization Association of Connecticut where all directors of Day Hospitals could meet to exchange the latest information on the most effective treatments of their patients.

I often told my immediate supervisor about what I had done at the program or about the work I was doing with other Day Hospitals in Connecticut. He seemed strangely uninterested. He ignored any treatment suggestions I made at staff meetings and usually laughed when I spoke caringly about some patient for whom I was concerned. If I thought that a patient was overmedicated, he disagreed without even seeing the patient. He, himself, would often talk about patients in the most pejorative ways, and I found myself being openly critical of his seeming heartlessness.

He didn't believe that I should openly tell patients that I had once been depressed and that I had gotten over it. He didn't want me to hug patients or to touch them in any way. He told me I had to wear "professional" clothing (instead of the dungarees which I usually wore in order to make my welfare patients feel more equal), and he was furious with me for daring to use ordinary "street language," including swearing with patients. A year-long battle ensued in which I received a number of memos on my treatment methodologies in spite of the fact that these methods continued to be effective and beneficial for the patients who received them.

I decided to confront this misunderstanding by running an inservice training program at the Mental Health Clinic so that my supervisor and my other colleagues would see the obvious advantages of becoming more humanistic and *human* with patients. I believe, and still do, that acting as if the therapist is superior to the client, or some kind of mentally healthy God, is not only bad manners, it is downright psychologically inappropriate and unhealthy.

My supervisor did not even attend the inservice, but I'm certain he must have heard how well-received the presentation was from the other therapists who were there. Instead, I was sent a memo ordering me to operate the Day Hospital in a "traditional manner, employing proven behavioral techniques." I wrote back that I would refuse his order in the best interest of the patients. He fired me.

Over 60 letters of outrage flooded in from patients, psychiatric professionals, other paraprofessional workers in the community, and the relatives of the patients whom I had successfully treated. This had no impact on the department of psychiatry, and I remained unemployed.

I made up my mind to do two things: to go into private practice and to study more psychotherapy. I wanted to choose effective therapists with whom I studied, and I found workshops and training programs by some of the finest Gestalt practitioners in the country. One of these, Laura Perls, was actually the co-founder of Gestalt therapy. Little did I know at that time that I would eventually dedicate a part of my life to being mentored by her. I also studied every book I could find on Gestalt therapy but kept myself open to other possible integrable theory bases as well. I took over four years of psychodrama training. Eventually, I entered a doctoral program in psychology at Union's Graduate School, studying biological, sociological, and psychological bases for behavior. This program was organized around a consortium of colleagues and universities. I was therefore able to study at a number of locations. No less than eight institutions of higher learning were sites for my advanced graduate studies. Finally, I entered a two-and-a-half year psychology internship with Laura Perls at the New York Institute for Gestalt Therapy. By June of 1981, I was well on my way to doing a preliminary search of the literature for my doctoral dissertation. On June 11th, my world collapsed.

By late August of 1981, I was very eager to leave the hospital and get back to my work with musicians using Gestalt therapy and to completing my doctoral work.

CHAPTER 8

The woman in 11 began banging the back of the bed with her head. "At least she had some neck movement," I thought.

A stream of curses flowed from her lips at her horrified mother and the nurse who was attempting to calm her down.

I heard the mother saying, "Lora. You've got to stop that Lora. Stop that right now. You aren't helping anyone deal with this thing."

Another woman's voice came through the wall. It was muffled and I couldn't hear what she said but she seemed to be struggling with the patient. The banging stopped. I imagined that the nurse was holding onto Lora's head and to keep it from smashing against the artificial-wooden headboard.

"Fuck YOU! Fuck YOU ALL!...Let go of my head you fucking cunt! Goddamn you all to hell...all of you." There was more banging. The nurse must have lost her grip on the flailing ball of hair.

"Oh Lora. How could you say those things to these people. They are just trying to help you. You've got to get better, darling. You know we all love you and want you to get better." The mother was talking to her possessed daughter. I thought of the mother from the movie, *The Exorcist.* I wondered if a priest would help. Visions of a holy water font suddenly sprang into my head and just as quickly I shrugged them off. I climbed into my wheelchair and headed out of my chamber. In the hallway I could still hear the shouting.

"Fuck your love! Can your fucking love bring back my body!! My body is dead!! Goddamn you all to hell!" Lora was screaming at them now. "Get the fuck out of my room you cunts!"

Both the nurse and mother went out into the hall. They looked totally defeated. The mother had dark, grey circles under her reddened eyes. She had done a lot of crying, worrying, and praying in the last few weeks. She looked unkempt, as if she hadn't changed her dress in several days.

The nurse was just feeling exasperated and furrowed her eyebrows as she stopped to look at the mother. They both paused for a moment to notice me pushing my wheelchair up the hallway.

"Mr. Gagnon. Maybe you can talk to Mrs. Broder—Mr. Gagnon is a counselor," the nurse said aside to the mother. "He can maybe tell you about what your daughter is going through." Turning in my general direction. "Do you mind? Would you talk to Mrs. Broder for a minute?"

Looking and feeling eager to do something meaningful, I perked up. "Sure. Hello Mrs. Broder. I heard what happened to Lora. God, but it must be very hard for you and her to deal with this injury."

"Oh, Mr. Gagnon..."

"John," I interrupted, feeling a great surge of compassion. I rested my hands on the dusty, scratched rubber of the large grey wheels as I had so often done.

"John... You have no idea what we've been through. Poor Lora. She's so angry. Is there any way to stop her anger? I don't think I can take much more of it. It is so horrible!" She averted her gaze.

"Well, Mrs. Broder, Lora is going through a natural stage in her grief over the loss of body function and feeling. Usually when someone loses something really important or a loved one they go through a grieving process. The first stage is denial, that is, trying to make believe that nothing happened at all." I watched her for some sign of understanding. She looked back at me. I thought that I could see the glimpse of light behind her dark brown eyes.

"I see what you mean," she said, nodding. "Lora was very quiet for so long. It's like she didn't want to see what had happened to her."

"That's it," I said as I casually rolled my wheelchair over to the side of the hallway to allow two orderlies to push by with a patient on a battleship gray, metal gurney. "And the second stage of the process is usually anger. Of course, the anger is in proportion to the degree of loss." I pointed down at the bandaged stump on my left side. "In my case, for example, I felt a great deal of anger and now I'm mostly feeling sad. With Lora, the amount of loss was huge, don't you think?"

"Yes...yes it is." The mother looked down at the floor as tears welled up in her eyes and she began to cry. "I love Lora so much. How could this bad thing happen to her? She's so young...and so...innocent. How could God have punished her like this?"

I hesitated for a moment, felt confused, but spoke anyway. "I really don't believe that God punishes people like that. I think that God is here to help us in times of terrible loss and difficulty. I just think that bad things happen to people at random. That doesn't lessen the amount of pain you feel, though." I then felt momentarily embarrassed about trying to preach to her about something as vague as God. She didn't seem to notice. Instead, at this last statement, the mother sobbed heavily and pressed her hands against her face. She couldn't see the tears on my cheeks. She wouldn't realize my empathy for her daughter. After a while she spoke.

"Do you think you could see Lora? Would you help her with this…this *grief process*?" her face pleaded with me.

"I'd be willing to see Lora, but only time will really help her with the grief. In the meantime the best thing that you can do is to accept your own pain and Lora's anger. Both of you have lost a lot." She began to cry again while nodding her head.

"Thank you, Mr.…I mean, John. Thank you. Please help Lora. O.K.?"

"I'll talk to her." I smiled up at her and when she nodded and turned to leave I sighed heavily and turned the chair toward the entrance to my room. I passed through the doorway and went over to the side of the bed where the black, mottled guitar case stood. I had played guitar since college. As I looked at the guitar I realized that it might serve as an opening to spending a little time with the young patient next door. I balanced the case across the arms of the chair and wheeled back out and down to her room. At the opening I leaned over the top of the case and knocked on the door. "Hello? May I come in?"

"What? Who the fuck are you?" a demonic voice croaked from somewhere in the direction of the bed.

"I'm in the room next door. My name is John and I thought I'd stop by and say 'hello'."

"You play guitar?" She couldn't move her body but her head was propped up on the pillow and she could see me well enough.

"Yep. I sometimes play by myself to relax. Want to hear something?" I wasn't sure if this was the right thing to say, but it was all I could think of at the moment.

"No. I just want to…" She lay very still, very quiet. Her face betrayed the terrible torment seething inside, however.

"Wishing you could die?" I interrupted her thinking.

"Yes. How the fuck did you know?" She stared up at the ceiling and bit her lip.

"I felt like that too. It's better when you stay pissed, though. There's more energy in being pissed."

Feeling affirmed a little her voice changed, grew stronger. "I am pissed. PLENTY! But my mother and the nurses here…they don't understand. They keep trying to stop me from hating."

"You've got every reason to hate, Lora. You got something to be plenty angry about."

"Shit!" she exclaimed. "I DO! My whole life is fucking ruined. What kind of life is there for me now? I don't have any feeling and I can't move my hands or my legs. There's nothing left for me to do. I never thought something like this would ever happen to me. I feel fucking awful." Her lips trembled and she bit down on her lower one again. Her eyes darted nervously to my face.

"It's O.K. I won't go away when you feel pissed. You can be as angry around me as you like," I returned instinctively.

"God bless you," she said, her eyes trying to see my entire length. Suddenly her face changed. "God! God? If there *is* a God! FUCK GOD!" She yelled out and then fell silent.

Her breathing was erratic but she lay quiet for a long time. Every few minutes she would glance over to see if I was still there. I hadn't moved at all. I simply sat there and looked at her with a lot of compassion and acceptance. Finally, after what must have been over 15 minutes she vocalized, "Shit, it's good not to be abandoned for being angry at God."

Another very long time passed. She sniffed hard and said, "I'd like to hear a song now. Do you know any new stuff?"

"Do I look *that* old?" We both laughed.

Besides visiting Lora each day and sometimes playing a song or two for her, I found other ways to feel useful on the unit. I got myself a "job." I was allowed to do vital signs for the nurses. Each morning I'd strap on my wrist watch, wheel down to the nurses station and pick up a stethoscope, a pad, and an electronic thermometer with disposable plastic mouth pieces. From there I'd go to each patient's room in the Rehab Unit and take their pulse, count respirations and do a blood pressure. I had done a lot of these as a lab technician in Griffin and St. Vincent's hospital in the days when lab technicians also took vital signs for donors who came into the blood bank. I was delighted with the "job."

By late morning I was usually occupied with physical therapy and a trip down to the whirlpool bath. There they would unwrap my thigh bandages, soak me in Betadine solution for an hour, and then spread Silvadyne Cream over the open areas of raw tissue. The procedure would end with a redressing of the infected area.

In the afternoon I worked on my search of the literature for articles relevant to my doctoral research and dissertation. Things felt almost normal again—almost normal, but not like being at home.

The Medichair Ambulance Company had a service which some patients on the rehabilitation unit could use with doctor's orders. It was expensive but worth more than every penny of it. On Sunday, August 23rd,

I was allowed to make a visit home in my wheelchair.

At 10:00 a.m., two strong medical technicians in forest-green uniforms, pushed my chair up the ramp into the van and locked it securely into place. I looked eagerly at the outdoor sights as the van took me away from the hospital. It was a beautiful day. The sky was blue and filled with storybook clouds…just like on the day in June when I went for a ride on my moped. I began to lose my initial aesthetic pleasure. My breathing got shallow and I got scared again.

On the highway I saw several large, shiny tractor-trailers. As they came by the van I burst into tears. I quickly put my hand over my mouth so the driver and assistant wouldn't hear me crying. I cried again as the van approached the tiny brown cottage. I had loved decorating it and considered it a real home.

Carolyn had not been fond of living in a rented house and had refused to do any gardening around it for the previous few years. I once told her that by investing energy into the garden she would make the house feel more important and like it *was* hers. She told me in the hospital that she was doing something around the house now and it did make her feel better about it. There, beside the steps was a flower bed where the dry dirt had been.

Carolyn and Isabelle came running down the steps and we hugged on the lawn before the two technicians lifted the chair up the four steps and over the sill into the living room of the tiny cottage.

The place looked the same. I had missed home. I didn't realize how much until now. I noticed the pewter cups on the mantel above the fireplace. I gazed at the books on the shelves near the couch and the large, colorful picture above. There were our riding ribbons and two of my antique guns hanging over the door to the hallway. My mother's lamp stood next to the couch, and my computer was still where I left it, on an end table. My eyes ate up the room. I feasted on all of the familiar objects, memorabilia and wood tones that I had called home for all of our time together as a family. I remarked wistfully, "The house hasn't changed at all…" and added after a moment's thought, "I have!"

Following the usual amenities, the two medical technicians left and we began to get to know one another again. The visits in the hospital were a kind of unreality. In this setting, the fact of the accident and its damage was unavoidable. I had "brought it home," literally. We talked animatedly for at least an hour, and then Isabelle went outside to give Carolyn and me some time alone.

I crawled down from the seat of the wheelchair and dragged myself across the rug to where Carolyn was seated near the fireplace. We lay on the rug together, holding onto one another as if letting go would make the other disappear. The sobbing was long and hard. I don't remember when we fell asleep.

We awoke in the late afternoon, wrapped in one another's arms. Somehow we had managed to pull a dark brown, fur blanket from the couch over ourselves.

I looked into Carolyn's grey-blue eyes and smiled. She returned the smile and then frowned. Her face became pained and she sobbed against my chest. When she stopped and Isabelle had come out of her room, I crawled back up into the wheelchair and waited for the arrival of the van. Within a half hour it was outside in the driveway. How short the visit had seemed. How long the time in the hospital had been. It took a great deal of effort to welcome the technicians back into the living room to let them carry my chair out of the house for the return trip to Danbury Hospital.

Monday night I got a visit from Bill. He was an old friend of mine from Southern Connecticut, and I hadn't seen him in a while. His mustached smile was broad when he saw me.

"How the hell are ya?" Bill's dark, Italian eyes twinkled.

"I'm O.K. How you been?"

"Don't get laid enough—you know, I never could understand why women put so much energy into guarding a damn hole—but otherwise all right," he laughed.

We talked over old times and caught up on all the happenings since the accident. Then Bill told me he had brought a present for me. He fished around in his jacket pocket and pulled out a marijuana joint. I felt amused by the idea but didn't take it seriously at first. It had been a number of years since I had smoked marijuana and now I was so drugged up I didn't think it was a good idea to try. After he had taken a couple of tokes, however, I gave in and took a long puff.

The smoke irritated my lungs and I coughed, but I welcomed the opportunity to escape reality a bit. As the next few hours went by, a number of interesting things happened. We finished the joint. That was the first thing. Then the nurse came in and announced that a patient on the ward had invited a belly dancer to entertain the patients and that she was going to wheel me down to the lounge. I looked at Bill as if I had just hallucinated the whole thing and he grinned back, "Hey... what the fuck!"

So there we were, stoned out of our minds, sitting in the lounge with a grown woman careening around the room and shaking her chain-covered belly at each of us in turn. The music was produced by a portable "ghetto blaster" which she had placed at one end of the room and by the tiny finger-cymbals she clanged together in rhythm to her undulations. At one point Bill turned to me and said, "This is some of the best pot I ever smoked! I got to find out where the hell Jim got this shit!" I laughed and nodded. The silly grin on my face was the only sign of how stoned I was.

When the dancing had ended and I was heading back to my room, another nurse approached to inform me that Fran and Alan Stave had come to see me and were waiting in my room. "Oh shit," I thought. I didn't want them to see me in this condition.

Have you ever gotten drunk as a teenager and then tried to sneak into the house, past your parents at the T.V. set without letting them know you're looped? I remember doing that as a kid. I spoke so clearly and distinctly that my mother thought I had taken leave of my senses. That's what Fran's face betrayed as I said, "Oh Fran. It is so good of you to come to visit me on this occasion of my hospitalization."

Several more uneventful weeks passed in the rehab ward. I continued to do my "job" and to counsel Lora. She had made a small amount of progress staying with her anger and was beginning to pass in and out of sadder moods when she and her doctor decided to move her to a rehabilitation hospital for spinal-cord-injury patients.

One morning I woke up, ate breakfast, took vital signs on the other patients and then wheeled up to Lora's room. It was empty. The bed was undone and she was simply gone. I felt badly that we had not had a chance to say goodbyes to one another. I returned to my room and cried.

Working with Lora had been very therapeutic for me. I hope it was of some help to her. I began feeling more confident each day that I had spent with her. My own grief, however, was persistent. I found it very hard to accept what had happened to *me* yet. I was filled with sadness. I wanted to be home.

A funny thing occured on the day of my discharge from the hospital. No matter how much I had wanted to go home, when the day arrived, I was afraid to leave.

"Institutionalization," I thought on Saturday, September 12th, the same day I called several stores to find out about getting a large, firm mattress for our water bed. Carolyn had already called the Home Health store for things like a trapeze over the bed, a transfer board for getting in and out of the wheelchair and a shower stool for the bathroom.

At my request, Tom, a friend of mine from down the street, had built a ramp from the driveway right up to the front door. I would be able to get from the house to my office in the garage. I could still work.

On Friday, September 18th, a few days before discharge I wrote in a personal journal, "I am so scared to go home. I don't know if I can go on with my life in a functional way. I feel insecure about doing therapy, about keeping my practice going, about my doctoral program. I'm even scared about trying to do computing again. I don't think I remember how to program anymore. I AM SOOOOO SCARED!"

CHAPTER 9

I went home on Monday. By the following Friday I had called 23 former clients, eleven of whom wanted to continue therapy with me; arranged all of the final details for the wooden ramp in front of the house and for another cement ramp up to the door of the office; notified Larry Huntley in the WesConn music department that I would be continuing my research on student musicians that academic year; started a physical rehabilitation schedule with a private therapist; saw the visiting nurse for my first of many weekly appointments; and called the Danbury News Times to tell them that they could write a followup article on my front-page accident of three and one half months before. I also had begun to take myself off of all of the medication on which I had been for months. I went through a slower, controlled withdrawal and within five weeks, except for an occasional sleeping pill, I was medication free. The next week I was seeing my clients on a regular schedule and had arranged for my friend Janet Swift to spend some daytime hours with me, especially around lunch time when I felt the most lonely and physically unable to do things. Carolyn was now working the day shift at the hospital and she looked more rested as she slept better during the night. I readied myself to work once again with musicians using the principles and methods of Gestalt therapy.

In October of 1981 I conducted the first session of my second year of research. Every Thursday night, one of the musicians from Western Connecticut State College came over to the house to pick me up and get me over to White Hall for the three-hour Gestalt therapy group.

John C. was a friendly, smiling fellow of 18 years who showed tremendous promise as a musician. As I began to work with him I encouraged him to play any piece of music he wished. John selected a rather lengthy Vivaldi duet of which John, of course, only played one part, the part for his instrument, the guitar. His phrasing was, at first, quite beautiful, his technique magnificent, but as John progressed, a slight tremor began to appear in his right hand. The music started to sound more and more choppy, less certain and less distinct. The music took on such a "nervous" quality that after a while I began to feel quite uncomfortable and restless listening to it. I stopped him from playing further.

"John, what's doing with you right now?" I shifted about in my wheelchair.

"I feel embarrassed that you stopped me." He looked rather sheepish.

"No, I mean: the music sounded...nervous...is the best way I can put it."

John leaned his guitar back against one of the metal folding chairs and folded his arms across his chest. "Oh yeah, I always get nervous when there are so many music critics around." His eyes darted around the group.

"So, for you this group is full of critics? Let's check this out. John, would you pick some people and ask them if they felt critical of you?"

John looked immediately at Brian, another guitarist. "Brian?"

"No...Shit...I'm always impressed with how well you play!" Brian sounded quite authentic.

"Do you believe him, John?"

"Yeah, I do..." He took a second look at Brian's face and then nodded. "Thanks Bri."

"Well, then, who would you pick next?"

"Stacey?"

She looked up with a tiny startled reaction. "God John, I think you're the best musician in this group. You just gotta stop getting yourself so nervous."

John nodded again, smiled and said, "How about you, Bob?"

Kidding at first, Bob replied, "You play rotten!" John and Bob both laughed at this. Bob then said, "No, seriously...You play much better than me. I envy your talent."

"Anyone else?" I queried.

"Jim?"

The burly percussionist straightened up in his chair. "Nope, I wasn't feeling critical of you. I just started feeling nervous for you when you were shaking a lot."

I began stroking my chin and nodded to Jim's last statement. I turned back to John. "So, what do you think about this critical bunch now?"

"They're not really critical of me. I don't get it."

"Do you know *who* is critical of you?"

"No, who is?"

"You are. You're the critic," I interpreted. "So let's have you own your critical self now. Would you go around the group and see if you can find anything at all to be critical of?"

Looking quite uncomfortable and sheepish again, John finally shrugged his shoulders. "You mean…actually say it?"

"No. For now it would be enough just for you to think it. O.K.?"

"Okay. That feels much better." John carefully looked at each member of the group. After a few moments of observing the first person, on John's left, a wide, sneaky grin appeared on his face. He repeated this with each member that John faced. When he seemed satisfied enough, he turned back to face me. "Okay, I'm done."

Already knowing his answer, I said, "Did you have any critical thoughts?"

"Oh yeah!" Again John gave me a broad grin.

"O.K., so now let's do this. I want you to play for us another piece, not the same one. You've already rehearsed that one. Only this time, I don't want you to start playing until you've taken a little while to be critical of each one of us…a sloppy shirt tail, messy hair, bad makeup…anything."

John smiled his understanding. Taking a good long time to go around the group, John seemed to find something about each person about which to feel critical. Each time John showed that grin he moved on to looking at another group member. Finally after looking at everyone, even me—and grinning—John began to play a different piece. It was quite complicated, but John handled all of the transitions on the fingerboard with ease. At no time did the music sound nervous, and after four or five minutes, the piece came to a firm, crisp end. The group spontaneously applauded.

"No shaking this time," I said with a Mona Lisa smile.

"Nope. I felt really powerful…in charge. It was like I was really important."

So when you own your criticalness and turn it outward, instead of back at yourself, you don't get nervous."

John nodded and then met my eyes. "But listen, I've got a recital this week."

"O.K. Do the same thing at that recital you just did here. Find something about the teacher to criticize: a zit, anything." The whole group burst out laughing at this possibility.

"Okay, I'll try it."

On the following week, John reported that while he was at first scared to do the assigned exercise, he finally managed to think up a dozen critical things about the teacher. John then played confidently until the last few measures when he became suddenly very critical of his own posture and the angle he was holding the guitar. At this point he began to tremble. In subsequent weeks, however, he gained a great deal of confidence by undoing his retroflected criticalness and by giving himself the permission to freely criticize others: teachers, audience, anyone. Eventually, even this energy began to change. After one concert before the holidays, John hugged me and thanked me for his lack of nervousness and his high level of excitement.

I remember my erstwhile mentor, Laura Perls, once saying to me that anxiety was the "flip side" of excitement. Anxiety also comes from the Greek word, *angustia* which means "to narrow or constrict." So by being self-critical, John had narrowed and constricted his energy. He became anxious. By freeing up this constricted energy, John was able to use the excitement in his playing. The results were impressive.

A 25-year-old cello player, Beth, was very clear that she wanted help with her performance. I learned that she had been a cellist for twelve years and had had three teachers so far.

A frail-looking woman, Beth seemed too weak to even lift the instrument, but she was surprisingly strong and agile when she positioned it with one hand. She sat back in the chair and rested the cello between her knees with the neck of the instrument up to her left shoulder. She began the session by playing a Bach Cantata. Her left hand trembled slightly (not just in the making of vibrato) as she played, and her body was not involved much in the music as she bowed. There was no apparent rhythmic relationship between her breathing and phrasing at this point. The music was plain and simple, devoid of mistakes but also markedly *dispassionate*. She stopped after completing one movement and looked at me, then quickly cast her eyes downward.

"I wasn't very good. My breathing is all off and I felt afraid of something. I don't know what it was, though."

"O.K., Beth, so you are aware of your breathing."

"Yeah, it's all off. David, my present teacher, has been trying to get me to work on it."

"I believe that there is a very important relationship, Beth, between breathing, movement, and phrasing."

She nodded and then clasped the bow tightly between her folded hands.

"Let me demonstrate that relationship." In spite of my confinement I began to move the wheelchair around the room. As I turned the wheel I either inhaled or exhaled as befitted the movement. While one arm was turning I occasionally gestured with my torso or free arm as in the ballet maneuver, *port de bras*. Some movements were begun with the audible exhale of breath, rests were accompanied with inhales and new "phrases" of movement again begun at the start of the exhale. When I finished I bowed at the waist. "There. How's that?"

Smiling, she replied, "Wonderful. That's it exactly."

"O.K., so play again this cantata and see if you can begin to experiment with breath and bowing so that you inhale with rests and move and exhale together."

She nodded and adjusted the instrument once again. This time she was clumsy at first but became increasingly more coordinated as the music progressed. The music was phrased at more appropriate moments, but there was still much holding back in terms of emotional expressivity. At one point her fingers began to tremble again and she looked a bit frightened. She ended.

"How was that for you?"

"Better...Much better...but...I experienced an interesting fear, a hesitation."

"What kind of hesitation?"

"Here..." She began to play the passage in which I had seen her fingers tremble. "When I make this transition..." As she demonstrated this, her fingers moved shakily from a position high on the neck to a place on the body of the instrument. It was clearly a difficult transition. "I'm afraid of something...of...falling off the fingerboard. That's it."

"So let's hear a little bit of this falling off. Play some music for me with a lot of difficult transitions and fall off of the fingerboard on purpose, O.K.?"

She smiled and then chuckled at the thought of this silly request but she played another piece during which she demonstrated many examples of falling off of the fingerboard. She laughed at times and her face became flushed.

When she finished, I queried, "How's that?"

She blushed all the more and fidgeted with her bow. "That was fun, but I can remember a teacher...Mr. J., who would be furious if I ever played like that." Suddenly a dark cloud passed over her face.

"If we could bring this teacher into the room and sit him over there..." I pointed to an empty chair. "What would your feelings be?"

"Scared!...I didn't like him very much. He was very strict and harsh with me." She began to shake.

"You seem frightened right now."

"Yes...and...um...I guess...angry too."

"I'm not surprised. So let's try an experiment. Let's imagine that Mr. J. is sitting right there on the bed, listening to you."

"Oh shit!"

"Oh shit, what?"

"He's so critical. I think he hated women." Her knuckles were white now as her left hand "strangled" the neck of the cello.

"What would he say or do to you right now?"

"After what I just played he would say..."

Interrupting, "Beth, would you show me by going over there and becoming him right now? Play him on the chair and speak to Beth."

She changed places and became the teacher, Mr. J. "That was awful! Terrible! You weak, feeble woman, you!"

"What do you mean by 'weak,' Mr. J.?"

"Uh...weak...sexually vulnerable."

A bit shocked, I recovered my composure and proceeded. "Sexually vulnerable?"

Beth returned to her own chair and answered. "Yes, like susceptible to being sexual and, therefore, weak. Unable to do the disciplined things a man can do."

"So you are not supposed to be sexual? You'll be weak if you are?"

"Yep." She separated her knees to replace her cello. "That's it." Her legs closed on this note. The cello remained by her side.

"Beth, now reposition your cello and play this piece again, but this time see if you can play it for Mr. J. with all the sexuality and passion you can put into it."

At first Beth seemed hesitant to try, but she adjusted the supporting leg of the cello, took her position and played. The music flowed easily and energetically with Beth breathing heavily throughout, *coordinated with her bowing*! The overall effect was positively beautiful. Finished and blushing, Beth looked at me again.

"Beautiful!" I applauded.

"Yes. Thank you. It was very good. I had no problem at all making the difficult transitions. I didn't even think of falling off the fingerboard and my breathing was right with the bowing. The phrasing seemed just right." She looked genuinely proud.

"So, when you don't obey this teacher's message and you, instead, play your music with your flowing sexuality, you don't fall off the fingerboard and play with better phrasing, with passion. Is that it?"

"Absolutely!"

Understanding the therapeutic moment, I concluded, "This seems like an important thing to remember."

While he was a guitar player, Tony's major was actually composition. During one group session, Tony asked if he could just work on an issue he was having in the area of composing new scores. I agreed, though I regretted that I wouldn't have a musical metaphor from which to initially make a diagnosis for the session. Tony took a chair opposite to me and brought along a brief case.

"All right, Tony, take out one of your musical compositions."

"I don't have any with me tonight." He looked immediately like he had already won some kind of competition.

"That's O.K." I felt undaunted. "Then let's imagine you have one with you."

Looking less pleased he mumbled, "Okay."

"Imagine placing it before you on the desk. Now look at this composition and constructively criticize it."

Looking down at the school-chair writing table, Tony took a long time trying to imagine the score. After five minutes or so I said, "It's O.K., Tony. You don't have to do this perfectly."

He immediately brightened and began. "Uh…Okay…well…I know what's wrong with this composition. It's got too many ideas at the same time. It's too loose. It's like I got to get all my ideas down on paper at once and I can't get them out fast enough."

Placing another chair opposite to Tony I said, "I'd like you to imagine that the part of you that composes loosely and tries to put everything down at once is over there."

He nodded. "I get it."

"Now tell him what you think of his composing."

"Well, you are too scattered. You don't have any compositional discipline. You are unable to put down one idea at a time and you work too fast. You try to get it all down and you end up going in circles. You have to…um…slow down. Get your ideas organized."

"O.K. Now change chairs and become the errant composer part."

As Tony moved over and sat he actually looked younger to me. "But I have to express myself. I've got to get my ideas out and down and when you have so many ideas…so many ideas to get down…I've got to express myself!"

"Now you're talking in a circle. So, switch chairs and let's hear what the other part wants to say."

Back at the "critical chair," Tony said, "That's right. You're doing it right now…going in circles. You try to express an idea and then you just end up repeating yourself because you're in such a hurry…so, slow down, will ya?"

"Switch."

As the composer, Tony looked hurt. "You're right, but when I try to do it your way, then you say nothing is good enough and when I try my best, I feel lousy that my best is not good enough for you. I mean, I've got to create and I try to slow down and do it your way. I've just got to get it down…"

"More circles," I interrupted. "Change."

"Yeah, see. You keep creating the same thing again and again."

"So here is your conflict, Tony. On the one side there is a creative child who tries to do eight million things at the same time and ends up only repeating himself. On the other side, you are so critical that when he slows down, you find nothing that he does good enough."

"That's right. I mean—what he does is workable—but I just don't think it's any good."

"Change chairs and respond to this."

Tony moved quite rapidly this time. "It is good enough! It *is* good enough but you criticize me so much I end up scratching it all out and never write anything." His mouth pursed into a child-like pout.

"I have a suggestion for you both. Ask...," I said addressing Tony as composer, "him to let the 'workable' stuff stay long enough for another opinion."

"Yeah, let this 'workable' stuff alone and let me hand it in to my composition teacher."

"Now change and experience how this idea sounds."

As the critic, Tony responded, "Well...It would be a reasonable test of what you're doing...I'll do it!" His face immediately brightened.

"O.K. So, your homework this week is to write a thoughtful, careful, workable piece of music...not 'great' or 'perfect' music, just workable. Then...would you hand it in...in to your composition teacher?"

He smiled. "Yep. I'll do it."

I ended the session with him by telling Tony that this issue might come up again in the same or a different form but that I'd be happy to work with him each time on this "composition issue." Actually, I realized that it was an issue about perfection. He seemed pleased with his progress after this. His teacher remarked that his scores were "quite good" and actually suggested his submitting some of them to a music magazine.

CHAPTER 10

Sissy Spacek was on the screen. The movie was *Coal Miner's Daughter*. I liked Sissy Spacek and had a crush on her for years. The wheel chair hurt quite a bit. I had been sitting all day long with clients and had just finished working in the kitchen (doing dishes) from the chair. My tail bone was getting sore and I momentarily thought about a decubitus. I thought longer about how sweet it felt to be home again, back to working with clients, and I was feeling quite proud to be off of all addictive medications, especially the pain killers.

The T.V. caught my attention again. Carolyn had cable installed just before my discharge from the hospital. With two home movie channels, a total of 37 channels were now available for day-long viewing. Isabelle was, like a normal nine year old raised on TV, quite happy. She enjoyed the variety and the possibility. I, on the other hand, was a little worried. I liked watching movies without leaving the house. I could easily get "drawn into" the TV, trance out and spend my entire evening, like Chauncey Gardner, "just watching." This passive couch potato was not the kind of person I had always been. For the previous five years I had led a very active, energetic, and physical existence. Something would have to change.

The physical therapy had been coming along. The therapist was tough with me. Louise, or "Lou" as she liked to be called, was like a little drill sergeant. I would bitch and moan about the pain I was experiencing, but she insisted on keeping me involved in daily exercises to try to stretch the

Achilles tendon in the pronated right foot. I was sometimes lax on doing the exercises but mostly kept up with the schedule that Lou gave me. By October I had gotten used to standing up on my artificial leg although I had bled pretty badly from the foot graft sites when I began trying the leg out in September.

I had already attended a horse show at Janie Starbuck's Stepping Stone Farm and had taken some great photographs with a new telephoto lens I had bought. The lens gave me the feeling of being more mobile than I was—that I could cover greater distances. Carolyn carried my chair around on a rack that went on the back of the car's trunk lid.

Sissy Spacek smiled sadly at me from the screen. "Something is not right tonight," I thought. My ass ached and my body ached to...to do what? Wasn't I doing enough already? I had a pretty busy schedule and enough books to read to occupy my mind. "I want to be on my feet again," I thought. I vowed that evening during *Coal Miner's Daughter* to make some kind of change in my evening time schedule. I had to play some kind of sport again.

Volleyball was an adult, evening event held at Ridgebury School every Tuesday, and Carolyn and I used to play sometimes before the accident. We decided to do it again.

I used to be pretty good at playing the net. My height was my main advantage, and I could customarily spike the ball well if someone "fed me." In the wheelchair, I was only about four feet tall. I decided to stay in the back court and my team let me do most of the serving. It was invigorating. I enjoyed trying to apprehend where the ball was going to land if it came into my area. I would quickly flip the wheels on the chair and lean way over to pop the ball up to where someone else could make the set up at the net. We did pretty well together, and I remember the exhilaration of our first win.

The evening we won I made one play by actually diving out of the chair onto the ground. I just barely got under the ball and it was still in play as I crawled back to my seat. There would have to be more of this activity. It was helping tremendously with my damaged self-image. That evening when I got home I even felt courageous enough to make love with Carolyn.

I sat at the edge of the converted waterbed for quite a while mustering my determination to feel as normal as possible. Carolyn first admitted that she felt a little frightened of my appearance. She also didn't want to hurt me by "moving in the wrong way." So there we were. Timid, concerned, and repulsed. With a great deal of talking, patience, and compassion, however, we felt like we could try. In spite of our attempt to comfort and support one another through all of the vulnerable and timid feelings, we were pretty insecure that evening. I was downright impotent.

As the weeks went by and I became a bit more agile on the artificial leg, Carolyn and I got more and more comfortable with one another. The love making became more regular and I lost my impotency. At first it was not easy because my mind kept talking to me throughout the foreplay. It kept reminding me how I looked. It reminded me that I was impotent and would probably continue to be impotent for the rest of my life. I kept remembering the part of the course I had taken at Rutger's Medical School on human sexuality that dealt with sex therapy. It recommended that one not focus on performance, so that's just what I did. I allowed myself to *not have an orgasm*. The paradoxical permission was sufficient to overcome my impotence by the third or fourth week of our trying. It was also helpful to remember that we were there (in bed) to pleasure one another, not to demonstrate any kind of sexual accomplishment.

In November an aunt of Carolyn's told me about a program that was sponsored by the 52 Association, an organization dedicated to helping handicapped persons get back into sports. She told me about a skiing clinic they were having in December at Stratton Mountain in Vermont. I called the organization, received the application in the mail, and signed up as a handicapped beginner. As the day approached, I felt a great deal of insecurity about my ability to ski again. I had never been a very good skier to begin with: I often fell down and was never able to keep up with Carolyn or ski any kind of difficult terrain. Reluctantly, but with a desire to win back my ability to exercise, I drove the car alone up to Stratton Mountain.

The morning was cold, and there was quite a bit of snow on the roads in Vermont. I had never skied at an actual resort before and just the thought of this was a bit intimidating. The sign for Stratton Mountain loomed before me. I slowed the car and turned into the parking lot, the snow crunching loudly under the tires of the car, and followed the signs for the 52 Association. I parked in one of the "handicapped" spots about 30 yards from the front door and slid off the seat onto the cold, snappy snow. My artificial leg did not fit very well and already my stump hurt from depressing the clutch as I drove. Also, I was not very stable on slippery surfaces. I took a deep breath of the brisk air and said to myself, "Here we go!"

Four collapsable dining tables had been set up for registration. Seemingly contented handicapped people sat untroubled behind them. My leg hurt and I was limping. I approached the first table uneasily and asked information.

The sign-up was quite effortless. Everyone I met was very helpful and friendly, and I found that I would be rooming with two other guys in a very comfortable condominium with a fireplace. It all sounded quite agreeable, but there was one little thing that bothered me. I wasn't used to seeing so many amputees in one place. All of these people had one or both legs or an arm missing. It actually felt disgusting and repulsive to me. I didn't like admitting this to myself. I liked even less the idea that *I was one of them*!

With my luggage stacked by my bed and a schedule for skiing instruction in the morning on my bed, I cleaned up for supper and the wine-and-cheese get-together that was planned for the evening.

I met one guy at dinner with whom I got into a conversation. We mostly said things like: "How'd you lose yours?" and that sort of thing. I really don't remember much about him except that he had been struck by a car while riding a motorcycle and had won $50,000 in the law suit that followed. He bought a new Datsun, 280-Z with the money and was partying on the rest. It made me think of the suit which we had against the trucking company of the driver who hit me. Then I forgot all about it as the "mixer" began.

It was incredible how timid and shy I felt with all these handicapped people around. I didn't like to look at their losses. I didn't like to feel mine again. Within a half hour, however, this feeling began to fade and was replaced with a different feeling of strength, camaraderie and support that I hadn't known before. "What an assortment of strong, capable people," I thought. Survivors of Viet Nam, dozens of accidents, cancer and congenital defects, this mass of brave humanity was able to instill in me a sense of courage that I didn't know was possible. I felt totally and completely *whole* with them. It was something that I just couldn't feel around "normies" or T.A.B.'s (temporarily able-bodied people), as we sometimes called them. Doctors, lawyers, farmers, businessmen, white- and blue-collar workers of all types were represented in this group of "disabled" persons. Somehow, together, we were not disabled. We could do things. We could overcome disabilities and go on. I felt much more confident about trying skiing by the end of that evening. I went to bed and slept peacefully.

After a good breakfast of eggs, flap-jacks, fruit, and coffee, I went to the rental shop to get fitted for my equipment. Many amputees would have to learn how to ski with only one ski and two small skis attached to the ends of Canadian crutches. I would get the "flip skis" as they were called, but I would have to ski on two legs since there was so much damage to my right foot that I still could hardly move the right ankle. I remembered that I hadn't asked my doctor if I could go on this trip, but that didn't matter to me. I wanted to ski.

It took me at least a half hour of pushing and huffing and struggling to get myself up to the top of the bunny slope where the beginners were waiting for instruction. The instructor, a sturdy, smiling black man by the name of Billy Demby, was leaning on his regular ski poles. "Good grief, a normie instructor," was what came to mind. After giving some of the basic moves and suggestions for turns and after everyone had gone their turn down the bunny slope, arriving safely at the bottom, Billy turned to me and said, "You're next. Just push off and make one turn to the right." I felt petrified. I couldn't seem to move. My legs ached and I wanted to get out of this death-defying act I had been crazy enough to agree to. I decided to play on his sympathies.

"I'm an amputee, for God's sake. This is hard for me." I hoped he would excuse me from trying. Instead he simply shrugged his shoulders, and turning gently on his skis, made a series of gorgeous turns down to the bottom of the slope. When he arrived with the rest of the students he turned up to face me.

"I'm a double amputee," he yelled. There was no more complaining from me for the rest of the week.

On Friday there was a race. It was a handicapped race and was set up by types of skiing styles (one or two skis, etc.) but it was just like looking forward to the Olympics. I was nervous. I was entered in the "four-track" division (two outrigger poles and two skis leave four tracks in the snow). I watched the three-trackers come down. They looked quite smooth. Then my division was announced. There were only one or two other opponents in this category but I was determined to get a good racing time. We went through the starting gate in the giant slalom course on an intermediate slope on Stratton Mountain. I had never before been able to ski an intermediate slope without falling. At the end of my run I was ecstatic to have completed the course without fault. I was even more ecstatic when at the awards that evening I found out that my time was the best in my division and that I had won the first-place medal. I felt like crying with joy. All the way home I knew that I was permanently changed by this experience and that it would inspire me to want more physical accomplishments in the future. When I walked in the door of the house I picked up the wheelchair, carried it out to the garage and threw it in a corner, *never to use one again.*

After winning the regional championship in downhill slalom at Jack Frost in February, I came home and tore down the ramp in front of the house. I used my bare hands to do it. I felt great. I still had a few phobias, however, that I wanted to work on next.

Whenever I saw a tractor-trailer I literally shook with apprehension. If one passed me closely on the highway I felt furious with the driver far in excess to any normal reaction I might have previously encountered. I decided in April of 1981 to "get back on the horse." I went to Cycle Ranch in Danbury and began shopping around for a motorcycle. I wanted one that was automatic, that is, would not require my having to depress a shift pedal on the left side. I found a Hondamatic 400 cc bike that filled the bill. I told Carolyn about my decision and she was horrified. She felt sick thinking that I might again risk being out on the road with a two-wheeled vehicle when I had nearly lost my life on the moped. I understood her reaction, but at the same time I knew what I had to do to feel safe on the road again. Also my phobic reaction had extended to riding my bicycle on the back roads around the house. I was terrified of being exposed. Carolyn told me that she might have to protect herself by withdrawing her love from me. That felt unpleasant, and yet I still knew in my heart that I had to get back on something that was safer than a moped but was like that two-wheeled vehicle. In May I received the Hondamatic and took it to the playground of a school where I practiced turns, stops, and so forth. I took the test for adding "motorcycle" to my driver's license two weeks later and passed. When I felt confident enough, I began to ride on small back streets in Ridgefield, and I always came home to park the motorcycle out of Carolyn's sight (as she had requested of me). One day I was ready for the big piece of therapy. I drove back over the same route that I had covered on June 11th, 1981. I rode through the pattern on Route 7 and remembered all of the parts of the incident. I then rode home, parked the bike out of sight, went into the office and screamed, off and on, for several hours. My voice was gone, my eyes puffy with the explosive crying, I stood up knowing that my fear was gone. I have ridden my motorcycle for the past seven years since and have never had any problem with it. I am very careful and I am no longer phobic.

The next thing that I wanted to do to deal with the accident was to do something about the dangerous intersection at Bennett's Farm Road and Route 7. I wrote letters to the State Motor Vehicle Department, state senators, other political persons and departments of the state. An investigation of the intersection was conducted, and despite the fact that there had been a number of fatal deaths at that exact location over the years, nothing was done to change the condition.

Next, there was my new-found sense of commitment to the issue of handicappedness. I began to find that more and more normies parked in handicapped places. Often, my stump blistered and bleeding from too much walking, I would have to hobble on crutches from the back of some parking lot because the handicapped space was occupied by someone who had simply parked there for convenience. I watched other disabled people wheeling their chairs down from a non-handicapped space, sometimes struggling unnecessarily to move over rocks or sand in the parking lot. I also watched some apparently normal people who parked in these state-regulated spaces and often asked them if they were handicapped. A few of them listened to what I said about the space being for disabled persons, and a few others were very nasty about it. I couldn't understand this.

One particular store owner parked his own car in the single handicapped space he had in front of his store. I asked him several times to please move his car. He always refused. I then began to call the Ridgefield Police to have his car ticketed. He ignored this sanction and continued to park there. Finally he painted out the space altogether so that there would only be normal spaces in front of his store. I called the State Department of Transportation about this and was told that by law as long as any store had fifty normal spaces it had to have one handicapped parking space. When I counted the spaces around the store I came up with approximately 40. I wrote letters to the local newspaper, who covered the story about the disappearance of the parking space, and the Town of Ridgefield then responded by ordering the owner, under an ordinance of the Town regarding handicapped parking for any store built after a certain year, to reestablish the space. He did and I felt like a very important step had been taken to preserve the rights of the disabled in Ridgefield. That same year the Town made many curb cuts to allow wheelchairs to move from the street up to sidewalks. Since 1982 I have always reminded normal motorists that they should not park in a particular space because it is needed by people in wheelchairs, etc. Sometimes I have been successful in raising their consciousness, sometimes they have ignored me altogether.

Lastly, I felt unfinished about the fact that there would always be accidents and always be persons in distress who needed help *before* official responders could get to them. I decided to develop an organization of "good Samaritans" who would be willing to stop for accidents and who might know what to do (or not to do) with an injured person. My life had literally been saved by *off-duty* EMTs before the ambulance arrived. Had these trained persons not been there, I might have bled to death before anyone responding could have saved me. I felt a strong obligation to return to others what had been given to me—my life. As I thought about this good Samaritan organization and its development, I discovered Ears React, a local group of good Samaritan individuals who use C.B. equipment to contact police and other emergency departments to help stranded or injured motorists. I learned how they evolved and how they were organized. I learned that Ears was not specifically trained to help with first aid, however. With the help of a few close friends, the Connecticut Emergency Service Association, as it was called, was organized in the spring of 1982.

We did not consider ourselves a responder organization at all, but rather, we would teach people the necessary first aid to help them help others. We would be a teaching organization in which the members would also be trained in helping others. Their stopping at an accident would be incidental and not the act of a radio-dispatched response team. Lieutenant Edward Schewe of the Bethel Police Department would teach all of the safety information about marking the scene of an accident with flares, keeping traffic away, etc.; Lieutenant Ted Peatte of the Ridgefield Fire Department would teach about how to handle car fires; I would be the director-pro-temp and teach about how to handle the fear and stress that accident victims suffer. We acquired a registered instructor of the American Red Cross, (also an auxiliary State Police Officer) to teach classes in first aid and CPR. I also wanted to know more about first aid, so I entered the EMT training program at the University of Bridgeport in May. I then notified the state department involved with non-profit organizations to register us with them and filed a not-for-profit status form with the IRS. I then met with Chris Gentile, the head of EMS in Connecticut, to be certain that we were not in violation of any state ordinances. He assured me that we were welcome as "Good Samaritans" just so long as we were never "radio dispatched." I also checked this out with Dr. George Terranova at Danbury Hospital. He was very interested in our vision of a civilian organization of persons who could provide first aid or CPR as required and wished me "luck."

Based on our fact gathering, we developed a constitution with bylaws to describe our organization and develop rules of conduct for the members. On May 22nd, Bristol Lettering Company began working on our sleeve patch, an eagle standing on a tire with the letters C.E.S.A. overhead on a field of sky blue. I was very happy with the way I was making lemonade from the lemons of only a year before. The Danbury News Times did an article on the C.E.S.A. asking for members. I also began to recruit from the ranks of other motorcyclists at a famous Sunday meeting spot called Marcus Dairy. Between the news article and recruiting we developed a founding membership of almost two dozen interested persons. Housewives, factory workers, business managers and others were among this group. The one unifying factor was their intense desire to help others.

On June 11th, 1982, the anniversary of the accident, I celebrated our success at a restaurant in Provincetown on Cape Cod.

The week I returned, I contacted Lieutenant Richard Dingee of the Ridgefield Fire Department and got permission for our members to be trained on their "Resusci-Annies" as part of the CPR practicum.

On September 25th I took and passed the state exam for EMT. At no time did any of the examiners notice that I was an amputee, and I may still be the only amputee EMT in the state system.

Afterwards I drove to a beach in Fairfield and looked out across the Long Island Sound. I cried with joy for how my life was turning around. By 1983 I completed my dissertation and oral defense, receiving a doctoral degree in psychology. I called my family from New York to tell them the good news. When I got home from the final review meeting, I found a bouquet of flowers from Carolyn on the doorstep. The note said simply, "Congratulations, John. You deserve good things."

Just before the holidays I finished working with a family. It was a long, difficult, and often painful bit of therapy and had gone on, with one year's hiatus, since 1980. I remembered how the case proceeded.

Fred was smiling at me. It was good to see the obvious happiness in his face; he had been depressed for such a long time. Fred was now 12 years old. I remembered how he was brought to my office in the summer of 1980 at the age of 10 by his mother, Alice Baker. He stumbled in the doorway like a reluctant dog on a leash. He was shy and miserable, and it did not take long for me to recognize the symptoms of childhood depression and low self-esteem, which his mother said was due to his "doing so badly in school." After most of the session with the mother talking for him, Fred was able to offer a few pieces of information about himself. He told me that he was also really poor at making friends and felt like a loner much of the time. He believed that nobody in school liked him.

Living in a town about 5 miles to the east of Danbury with his father Sam, stepmother Sharon, and brother Billy, Fred had been having more and more difficulty concentrating and paying attention over the summer prior to returning to school and actually seemed to be terrified of going back in the fall.

Fred told me that he was, indeed, "sad" because "other kids think I'm stupid...and they treat me rotten a lot." The first thing I wanted to check about his "stupidity" was whether or not Fred was dyslexic. His mother said that he was not and she gave me permission to contact the school system to get more information on him. When I received the report on his educational history, I didn't find any indication that Fred had a learning disability. He had been thoroughly tested and evaluated by the school system and by a children's hospital in New York State, and they decided that his problems were related to some kind of psychologically induced depression of long standing.

I remembered, however, what I wrote about Fred in my initial mental status examination.

> Fred presents himself as clean but unkempt, slumped, mildly anxious (appropriate to meeting me), distinctly depressed with a decreased variability of expression, decreased and slowed speech, somewhat eager to please and overly compliant. There is no sign of a specific learning disorder but I recognize various

> hesitations in sentence construction, attention deficits and defective motor coordination which, if not of depressive etiology, might be undiagnosed dyslexia.

I reserved this impression for a later time. My report went on.

> Affect and mood are consistent with depression; there are no illusions, delusions, hallucinations or other indications of a thinking disorder. Impaired level of consciousness is consistent with depression as is his difficulty with performing serial 7's and other tests of concrete as well as formal operational thought.
>
> Oriented in the usual spheres, Fred has no difficulty acknowledging his inability to perform well in school and also the inability to develop and maintain long-lasting peer relationships.

Fred blamed all of his problems on the aforementioned belief that other children thought of him as "stupid."

Fred described his relationship with his father as "good" and said that he "really liked Sharon," the stepmother. He said "things were o.k." with his brother Billy, but he fidgeted a lot when he said this and I was sure that he was trying to hide a considerable amount of displeasure with his brother. I felt a bit perplexed when I started to do therapy with Fred. I decided that I wanted to see him in his natural setting. I wanted to meet the "system." I invited the entire family in for therapy around Fred's difficulties. I met the members of the Westerly household as well as Alice Baker at that time. Various members described Fred as being a "sensitive kid" who got along well with his parents and stepmother, but occasionally fought with his brother (as expected). I was told that Fred loved animals and that he had been on visitation to see his mother (joint custody) on a biweekend basis. All members concurred that Fred appeared depressed and had a very low self-esteem. There was a lot of tension in the room as these various people talked to me. I sensed quite a bit of unspoken feelings from all of the members of the family system, but I knew that I had to build a relationship with them all before I could confront this fact. After a few sessions, I asked the family's permission to contact the school social worker.

Mrs. Ramon called me on the phone to say that Fred had been becoming increasingly frustrated as he progressed through school. As teachers' expectations for academic achievement increased, Fred was less and less able to keep up.

I decided that I would organize my therapy treatment plan in such a way that I could see Fred by himself and also see the whole family system in another session that same week. Fred was reticent during our first sessions together, but during the family sessions it became increasingly clear that the mother, Alice, saw herself as clearly outside of the parental system and not part of Fred's life in any meaningful way. I remembered trying to keep the group discussions at levels that were appropriate to adults as well as to the children. This often required translating what one member of the family was doing or saying to the other members. I employed several styles of speech. The children became more and more interested in what was going on in the family as I did this, and by the second month they were ready to try something called *family sculpting*. This technique allows each member of the family system to arrange the other people in the room into a giant "sculpture." This metaphoric arrangement often tells a great deal about the family and the dynamics within it. I was also interested in trying to help include Alice in the systemic structure. In the first sculpture, no matter who made up the family system, Alice was often placed or placed herself as far away from the other members as possible. I encouraged her and the Westerly family to try different arrangements of the sculpture to see what that would be like. After several months, Alice reported feeling much safer with the system and seemed to develop a special closeness with Sharon, who was showing signs of her pregnancy with Sam and Sharon's first child together.

In the individual sessions with Fred, I explored the ways in which he related to his peers. I role-modeled ways to talk to other children by greeting him every session as if we were just meeting for the first time. He would always chuckle over this imaginary play between us, but soon he was learning ways of saying friendly things to me when we met. He told me that he was "beginning to make some friends at school." I also did some direct coaching.

I gave Fred advice about things he could say to kids who didn't like him and who tried to insult him. He liked talking about these things and seemed to relish having some new ways of relating that might increase the likelihood that his peers would accept him. He would come back session after session saying that he tried the things that I was teaching him. He showed obvious pleasure at deflecting an insult and feeling o.k. about himself when he did. He began to feel more in control of his life. Fred became happier in sessions and even laughed over silly jokes that we made up between us. Always, however, there lurked in the background the poor school performance that threatened to keep Fred in the role of "stupid kid" in his class.

As his depression improved and Fred reported "feeling a whole lot happier," his school work did not improve. I decided to work with him on his verbal as well as written skills. Within a few sessions, it appeared that he was having a great deal of difficulty arranging words in the correct order in both areas.

I called the school psychologist, Dr. Ann Berkeley, and advised her to readminister a WISC-r, Bender Gestalt, WRAT-r, and TOWL to explore the likelihood of dyslexia. Following her testing of Fred on October 8th, 1981, she reported to me, the parents, and the school that he was "indeed learning disabled with an above normal total I.Q. but with verbal and nonverbal discrepancies as well as scatter on math questions indicative of a sequencing disorder." How everyone had previously missed diagnosing him was beyond me. I was amazed. The family was appropriately furious.

By November of 1981, it was clear to all of us that much of Fred's poor self-esteem was the result of his missed dyslexia and the way in which teachers as well as other students responded to him. There was also some indication that Fred was deeply concerned about the feelings in the family system and that he definitely wanted to see his mom and dad achieve some kind of peaceful resolution of their nonverbal hostilities. As Fred put it, "Mom and Dad don't say they don't like each other, but I know they don't."

Employing a great deal of denial, the family system only talked around the anger that they had for one another. There were some indications that Billy supported his mother and that Fred was trying to be a peacemaker for the whole group. Alice and Sam said that they were still angry about the "hurt of the divorce" but denied that there were any other negative feelings. As time went on, Sharon and Alice seemed quite friendly, and Sam and Alice were able to talk somewhat cooperatively about their children. Finally, the family system as a group told me that they had resolved their conflicts. I didn't believe this and told them so, but they indicated to me that I was mistaken.

In his individual therapy, Fred told me that he was feeling "just great" knowing that he was not stupid but that he had a learning problem, which he nicknamed "flip-flop." Fred knew that teachers were acting differently around him, and he also felt better about dealing with the other children in his school. He appreciated my teaching him some social skills for dealing with peers to whom he was attracted as well with those peers who gave him trouble. "I'm not stupid!" he said. "I just have a flip-flop problem and I get mixed up. I know how to tell the kids now, too. Thank you."

Fred was placed with Mrs. Pauling, a special education teacher, although he was eventually placed with someone with whom he felt more comfortable.

As the system was completing therapy, Tim was born to Sharon and Sam, and sibling rivalry was handled with a minimum of difficulty. The adult members and children of the family accepted Tim and integrated him easily into their system. As therapy came to a close, I recognized the tremendous allegiance that Billy seemed to show for his mother, and I suspected that he actually wanted to leave the Westerly household and live with her. This later proved to be correct.

I was also suspect about the unexpressed hostility Billy had toward his father and indicated that in some future session, he might wish to address this. We ended this span of therapy by March of 1982.

I called Alice and the Westerlys a few times to follow up after they completed therapy. I found out that Billy did, in fact, take up residence with Alice in September of 1982. He seemed to adjust to the new living arrangements rather well. The Westerly household reported missing Billy but wanted to respond to his need to be with his mother for a while. They grieved his absence appropriately. During this time, however, Alice developed a rather serious herniation of two discs of the spine, eventually requiring surgery and long-term bed rest. She got around with great difficulty and experienced a great deal of pain from another herniated disc that might yet require surgery. Billy had to deal with his mother's convalescence and in many ways took over as the little "man" of the house in spite of the presence of Alan, a friend and housemate to Alice who lived with them.

In March of 1983, I was again contacted by the Westerly family to inform me that Fred had been accused of stealing toys from a younger child. Parents of this child had called the Westerlys to inform them of this, and Sam, Alice, and Sharon were very worried that Fred was either developing a bad habit or that he was behaving in such a way that the other child's parents were misinterpreting his intentions. "Maybe the little kid gave Fred the stuffed animal," they said.

I agreed to see Fred immediately and to see the family system as we had done in the past. I arranged a session in which I would administer a kind of test to Fred that showed him pictures and asked him to tell me stories about them. In this way I could look at his sense of reality and judgement; his regulation and control of impulsive feelings; his continuing relationships with peers and the other members of his family; his thought processes; the kind of defenses that Fred tended to use to deny feelings; and the degree of control that he was feeling over his life. Before the day of this session, however, Alice and Alan (Alice's significant other) "interrogated" (he was a former police officer) Fred and "got him to admit that he was lying" about not stealing the other child's stuffed animal and that he had stolen a number of other toys from other children. In total, the children included a neighborhood boy who apparently "started it" by stealing a brand new baseball glove from Fred (Fred took one of his schoolbooks and threw it away), a younger friend Michael from whom Fred took a toy gun, and an inlaw's son, from whom he took an entire set of Legos. I was told that Fred said he did these things because "they felt good and all the kids around school take stuff." Fred seemed oblivious to any wrongdoing associated with his exploitative behavior, and the only thing that upset him was the punishment he would receive for being caught. This level of moral consciousness is consistent with a normal child of about 5 to 6 years of age. I listened to the report from Alan and then proceeded with the testing anyway.

Throughout the story constructions Fred made from the drawings, I found images of loss, death, suicide, and extremely harsh punishments for "doing bad things."

The first story told of Fred's continuing wish to perform well at school. In pictures 1, 5, and 8, fantasies of ghosts were described. When he talked of ghosts, things were "so much happier." I saw these as ghosts of Fred's childhood when his parents were together and Fred felt happier. Characters in these stories denied death (after all, they were ghosts), denied the death of relationships, and avoided relating to live people in the present. In some ways, Fred had gone dead and was refusing to relate to people in the present. This made sense.

In stories 3, 7, and 8, people were forced to destroy themselves out of guilt for what they had done. This was the first indication that Fred might feel guilt over his acts. In 4, 6, and 10, characters tried to comfort those in pain and to take responsibility for the pain or loss of others. This pattern of codependency first showed itself with Fred years ago during family sculpture and might, I believed, indicate his continuing need to manage the peaceful joining of his mom and dad.

His conception of the world was predominantly as a painful place from which one could only escape in work or by regressing to a lower level of development.

Relationships to others in his stories were full of rejection and abandonment. This was especially true when he described the characters as being "husband and wife." Fred seemed fixated on the breakup of his parents, and his acting out at that time in an inappropriate way certainly required that they come together to deal with his and their own problems.

In other stories, parents split up and friends "went away unless you took something to keep them there." This was certainly telling: Fred was obsessed with the fear of losing people. He had learned a lot about making friends in his first stint of therapy, but he had learned even more about loss from the breakup of his parents, whom he had loved so much.

Fred's stories told of worries over his adequacy as a boy, the pain of living, and the avoidance of this pain by flight into fantasy and untruth. I later learned from Sam that Fred had been chronically lying ever since I had seen the family in 1982.

The nature of anxieties Fred expressed or alluded to embodied abandonment or isolation in one form or another: not belonging to the school or group of peers, losing a loved one or oneself, a tremendous fear over *severe* punishment, and being unloved by the very people who should be nurturing him, his parents.

Fred's defenses included the use of fantasy and regression to lower-aged behavior. He also avoided painful truth and lied to me about his performance in school. I found out from the Westerlys that he was again doing poorly in his classes and might have to be held back another grade. Fred was using denial as his main defense, and when he lied he was able to convince himself that he was not as "bad" as he might be in the eyes of others, particularly his parents and his peers.

Fred's stories also showed that he felt like he had to "take care of others in pain." While this might, at first, have looked normal, it was actually a sign of codependency. Otherwise, when Fred did admit that he had done something wrong, he was very hard on himself, and his stories spoke of the unbearable punishments that awaited him.

Fred had become developmentally immature for his age, despite his obvious creativity and intelligence in making up his stories. He functioned morally and emotionally like a child of about 5 to 6 years of age.

In the development of a new treatment plan, I discussed this case anonymously with a number of colleagues who specialize in working with children. They indicated that dyslexic children sometimes have difficulty seeing right from wrong but that it certainly sounded like Fred was doing more than just missing cause and effect. They agreed with my conclusion that Fred wanted to rejoin the mother and father.

The new treatment plan consisted of seeing Fred on a weekly basis. I wanted to have him examine his beliefs about stealing from other children and also investigate the level of empathy that Fred could feel for the potential hurt he had caused to several younger children.

Since I had been successful in directly teaching him how to talk to other children in the past, I wanted to teach him about respecting the rights of others. I also wanted to help Fred learn impulse control and help put off the satisfaction of his wants. Since he certainly had not tried to hide his conduct or acted in a way that would have assured his not being found out, I was especially concerned with the manipulative value that his stealing had on others or the way that stealing served the function of keeping friends present, unable to leave him. My main interest, therefore, was in Fred's sense of loss and abandonment, his worries about present loss, and his secret need to get mom and dad back together.

I called in the entire family system again. It then consisted of Fred, Sam, Alice, Sharon, Billy, Tim (now a toddler) and Alan, Alice's friend.

In the first couple of sessions there was a great deal of appropriate anger expressed at Fred for his inappropriate behavior. Billy was also able to admit that he was afraid of Fred—that Fred might steal something from him. The system was encouraged to develop a strategy for monitoring Fred's behavior around other children until we could be certain that he was no longer interested in stealing from them. Everyone concurred and was encouraged to demonstrate his or her own understanding of this type of behavioral contract. Several weeks later, however, while his father was on a week's vacation, Fred stole another child's present at a birthday party. This was due to poor monitoring on Sharon's part and she readily admitted it. It was also, however, a way to get dad to return home prematurely. The family was able to see this but did not fully understand the significance of the stealing behavior as a way of getting people together.

In later sessions, an undercurrent began to develop involving groupings of members. This resulted in the formation of several alliances.

Alan and Alice took several sessions to inform the sytem what a poor father Sam had been and enumerated several examples of parental neglect. While I found Sam to be somewhat laid back in his parenting and Alice to be equally rigid and controlling, the comments attacking the Westerly family parenting seemed like a cover for a deeper conflict between Alice and Sam. Eventually what surfaced was that both of them wanted to fix the blame for Fred's aberrant behavior on one another. Sam attributed it to Alice's need to control and also to her "religious fervor." Fred was then able to admit his confusion over the "time Mommy told me that Daddy will go to Hell for living with Sharon before they got married." Fred also said he was terrified that he might go to Hell. Sam and Sharon were furious about Alice's "guilt trips." I proceeded very carefully at this point in the therapy.

On the one hand, I had to support the ethical beliefs of the mother while allowing for the possibility that both Sam and Fred were, indeed, "loved by God" and had the possibility to enter Heaven upon their respective deaths. For several weeks Alice rested all of her arguments upon the Bible and Alan agreed that "Fred's troubles came out of the evil in that house." Alice attributed Fred's lying and immoral behavior to Sam's "sinful conduct with Sharon in front of the kids." By this, she meant how Sam and Sharon had lived together before getting married. Billy joined in the alliance against dad by describing three separate occasions on which he thought that Sam was a bad father. My former belief that Billy had a lot of unfinished anger about his dad's divorcing his mother was correct. He agreed with his mother that "dad and Fred are evil" and seemed to delight in the power this gave him.

In one session Billy demonstrated how much power he wanted to have by demanding to know all of the "secret anger that daddy has for mommy." I denied him this power and immediately set up a session for Sam and Alice in which they could confront one another away from the rest of the devisive system. I got this idea from Ralph Welsh, another colleague, who suggested that I interrupt the system dynamics to allow the main combatants to fight things out. "Perhaps they will return to the larger system in a more allied manner," he said.

In the meantime, Alan announced that he did not want to return to therapy, that he was never "that close to Alice," and that he was actually "making plans to leave the house." I did not find him believable, but I did see an interesting connection between my isolating Sam and Alice and Alan's loss of his assumed position as a kind of cotherapist in the group. He never shared anything about himself, only passed judgments and made interpretations about the behaviors of others, especially Sam and Sharon. I encouraged him to see himself as an important part of the system since he coparented Billy and Fred when they visited Alice, but he was adamant about not continuing. This threatened to destroy the integrity of the larger system. I had to do some careful work now.

Alice announced that Alan would not return to sessions. I spent a couple of weeks just building new supports to restructure the family system to deal with the absence of Alan. I continued to see Fred for individual counseling and prepared the groundwork to gently expose the devisive alliances that had developed and that served no purpose but to continue the dislike of the original parents for one another. We began to make progress again. Fred became concerned about his former behavior and admitted in the family sessions that he had "acted like a little kid." He showed genuine remorse about his behavior and cried as he honestly recounted the stories of his stealing from the other children. Sam and Sharon were quite happy with this. Billy began to soften toward his brother and they became much better at playing together both in the Westerly home and when Fred visited Billy at his house. Alice said nothing and over a number of subsequent sessions seemed indifferent to Fred's confession or his changed attitudes and behavior.

Finally, Alice stated in one session that she "would not allow Fred to see me further," that I "was not the right therapist for Fred or for the rest of the family." Sam immediately confronted Alice directly, and no one tried to take sides this time. He said that she did not "have any right to try and control the therapy." He added, "I refuse to go along with your attempts to mess things up just when they're beginning to straighten out." Alice reluctantly came back for more sessions.

"What were we getting close to that caused Alan and Alice to want to drop out of the therapy?" I wondered. The breakthrough came in a couple's session between Sam and Alice. This occurred just before termination in November of 1983. The leaves were already well off the trees and it was time for something to die. It was the death of a relationship built upon lies.

Alice looked absolutely miserable as she sat on the couch in the office. Sam sat at right angles to her in an upholstered armchair. She did not waste any time.

"I have a terrible confession to make...." Her voice trailed off and she looked ashamed as she stared at a spot on my carpet.

"This must be rather difficult for you, Alice," I emphathized.

"Yes. It is very difficult...but I've got to say something or I'm going to go out of my mind." She hid her face in her hands as she wept, "Oh God...please forgive me for what I have done. Oh God...what *have I* done?"

"You want to straighten something out with Sam, Alice?"

"I must. I've been a terrible liar these past bunch of years. What a hypocrite!" Again she was overcome with remorse and cried for a while while shaking her head from side to side.

When she subsided I encouraged her, "Go on, Alice. Say what you can and go slowly."

"I've been a liar. Don't you get it? I've been a hypocrite all these years. I've condemned you, Sam, and degraded you in the eyes of your children and I was sleeping with Alan all of the time. I used my religion like a weapon to get you—God, but I hated you—but that was the wrong thing to do. I don't think you are a very good father, but it was wrong for me to make you look like such a sinner when I've been one myself." She sobbed wrackingly at this confession. "I don't want to lie any more. Oh God...I'm so ashamed, I've got so much to tell the children...to admit to everyone. How could I have done it?"

"You must have been pretty desperate, Alice, to lie like that. I know you were always pretty religious but you know it isn't any sin for you to love Alan like I loved Sharon." Sam was doing such a great job as supportive therapist that I just sat back and waited.

With a new rush of emotion, Alice cried, "Oh Sam, I am so sorry. I've been horrible and I did become a hypocrite, not for loving Alan but for making you into a sinner in the eyes of your children. That was wrong and I don't expect you to ever forgive me."

Well, Sam did eventually forgive Alice and so did the whole family once they attended enough sessions in which they could vent all of their various feelings: anger, frustration, disappointment, disillusionment and hurt at Alice. She did a very good job, with support, of withstanding the feelings of the family group. With the passing of time, they all came to accept one another.

Most importantly, Fred could become the normal, well-behaved adolescent he really wanted to be.

While my practice was taking up a good deal of my time, my passion for emergency services to others had not ebbed.

By the winter of 1983, the C.E.S.A. was in full bloom. We had trained over 24 people in first aid and CPR and were a viable body of concerned citizens. We did experience internal difficulties, however. We found no particular reason to meet on a regular basis except for training. When we finished with the first training group, there was essentially no reason to get together until we organized another refresher. The result was that only the original core of founders stayed together. Bruno Stroili (a sergeant) and myself were particularly interested in seeing the C.E.S.A. grow, but we didn't know how to make this happen. We often met to discuss this problem, as I discussed it with Ed Schewe and Ted Peatte, but we simply didn't know what to do. It was tabled until we could figure out how we might reorganize. By the summer of 1984 we decided to temporarily but officially disband the organization and notified everyone to that effect. We wanted to have a better plan for organization, but none of us seemed to know what that should be. Throughout all of this extra-curricular activity, however, I was still maintaining a strong private practice and working psychologically to heal others who were handi-capped. I was called upon to work with several handicapped patients at D.A.T.A.H.R. and to run a special group for spinal cord injured persons at We.C.A.H.R., two programs for the handicapped. Various emergency medical system departments in the state had called me to instruct them on how to handle persons suffering from alcohol or drug related problems or from mental disorders. I was busy and enjoyed the work. In addition to this, I decided to volunteer my time to one of the local police departments. In late August, I presented a plan to that department for helping and teaching the application of psychological methodologies to them. The chief was very interested and said that it was generous of me to volunteer my time, but that there had to be funds for me and he insisted that I be hired on some kind of stipend. When I later negotiated this with a department representative, we agreed on the amount of $2000.00 for all services and a 24-day on-call status for a one-year period. This seemed O.K. to me. I had been willing to do the job for no remuneration at all. I was assigned to Emergency Services. In the meantime, I got to apply my own EMT training to an emergency on a local highway.

I was driving east on Route 84 toward Newtown Health and Racket Club for some exercise. It was in the fall of the year. The trees were turning all shades of xanthrophil and tannin, and the smell in the air was the first smoke of fireplaces warming the hearths and hearts of the family. Sundown was coming a bit earlier now, and by 6:30 the skies were purple and orange splashes of paint against gray, stratocumulous streaks.

I have often seen cinematographic moments in which the speed of the film is increased to produce a slowed down action on the screen. Apparently, persons may experience a time distortion around certain events. At least, that is what the film artist hopes to produce. I had exactly that experience as I watched the dark green Chevy station wagon begin to cross the grass divider between the west- and east-bound lanes. I could see it well in the distance, perhaps as much as 3/4 of a mile away and it was moving, undaunted by the rough texture of the rutted, grassy surface, as quickly as it had been going moments before on the macadam highway. The driver of the maroon Ford in front of me did not seem to notice the approaching Chevy.

I watched without emotion as the green wagon rose up the sharply curved shoulder of the divider before becoming air-bound. The time was stretched out as the wagon, going perhaps 70 or 80 miles an hour, sailed slowly through the air and landed on the hood of the Ford.

Suddenly, the wiring in my head went into overdrive. Everything went back into real time. I slammed on the breaks, just avoiding the rear end of the Ford in front of me, which was now spinning to the left with the other car now sliding off of its hood and coming to a screeching halt perpendicular to the Ford, across the entire left lane.

Reaching down in front of the seat, I pulled up the emergency light which I had magnetically attached to the floor and stuck it on the slanted dash board of my dark blue Plymouth Reliant. I again reached down, this time to turn on the C.B. radio and adjust the frequency to Channel 9, the emergency channel allocated to occasions such as these which was monitored by both the State Police and Ears-React. As I pivoted my car across the left lane to stop all traffic behind the accident, I grabbed the microphone and pressed the talk button.

"Breaker 9, breaker 9...does anyone copy this emergency transmission?"

There was a pause and some static. I again repeated my call. "Breaker 9, breaker 9...any State Police or React people monitoring this transmission?"

"Roger," came on the crisp, clear signal. "This is Ears-React and we have your call."

"There has been a serious automobile accident on Route 84 East between exits 9 and 10, approximately one half mile after exit 9. Two vehicles have collided. There may be serious injuries. Advise police, EMS and a tow truck to clear the lane. Copy?"

"That's a 10-4, good buddy." He repeated the message and we signed off.

I threw open the car door and ran for the back of my car. Opening the trunk I immediately slung on the EMT belt with the stethoscope, shears, and window punch on it. I grabbed the orange jump kit and the black case containing the "D" cylinder of oxygen in the event that someone was going into shock.

Running as fast as my amputated leg could carry me I quickly triaged the situation. The man in the Ford was lying back against his seat and not wearing a seat belt. I could see him breathing in spite of the split lips and broken teeth—he must have hit the steering wheel—but he looked unconscious and I immediately thought of a neck injury and possible broken ribs or sternum. I would give him a high priority, but I needed to see the others in the wagon.

The six female passengers of the Chevy were already exiting. None of them looked seriously injured, although I could see blood on the front of the conservative dress of the driver. One of the passengers in the front was bending down and examining a large contusion on the front of her slightly bulging lower leg. Either the tibia or fibula was broken. This was not serious but I wanted her not to bear weight lest she pinch some important blood vessel between the broken bone ends. I identified myself as an EMT and asked her to please sit down by the large crowd of bystanders that was forming on the right side of the road. Another individual, a firefighter, had closed off the right lane with his car and emergency light. He was also setting road flares along the shoulder every 25 to 40 feet. I yelled to ask him if he was an EMT and he said, "No…wish I could help you, but I don't know the first thing about medical stuff." I handed some 4x4" gauze pads to the woman driver for the cuts on her face and got all six women, who turned out to be nuns, seated. All of the above had only taken less than 2 minutes to do. I did not want to waste any time on the less injured parties. I ran back to the man in the Ford.

As I ran up to the car I could see that he had not moved and was still breathing. I quickly grabbed the adult-sized Philadelphia collar I carried in my kit and yelled for an EMT or nurse. A woman already approaching the car said she was a nurse, and I asked her to hold traction on the driver's head while I put on the collar. She opened the rear door and climbed in behind him. Supporting his head from under the chin she lifted the spinal column into proper alignment while I velco-strapped the collar into place. Once completed, I grabbed my stethoscope and sphygmomanometer and asked the nurse to take vial signs.

She began pumping up the blood pressure cuff as I looked into the man's mouth to make sure that no blood clots or broken teeth could obstruct the airway. I pulled out a few shards of teeth, checked his breathing and then cut open the front of his turtleneck shirt with my shears.

The secondary survey of the chest proved to be almost negative. One area of the chest was quite red and the rib was indented beneath it. The broken bone was on the left side, and therefore, was unlikely a threat to any important arteries as, for example, in the liver which is on the right side of the body.

The nurse called out, "90 over 70. I did it three times just to make sure."

"O.K.," I returned. "Do you know how to use portable oxygen?"

"Yep. I've done it on transports."

"O.K., give me the full face mask with 4 to 6 liters-per-minute flow rate." She deftly opened the case, attached the tubing and set the flow rate while I covered the man's shocky body with my jacket. I continued the secondary survey to his legs to feel for any fracture of the femur. There was no swelling or discoloration when I cut open his pant leg. I took the oxygen mask as the nurse handed it to me and placed it on the victim's nose and mouth. His color was already starting to get a bit cyanotic. I slipped the elastic cord over his head to hold on the mask and wondered about the cause of shock. I reassessed the chest. Although I did not see anything at first, I now noticed that the front of the sternum, which had not previously shown any sign of injury, was now bright red. The man had stuck the steering wheel right above his heart. There could be some local bleeding around the heart or in the pericardial sac that was tamponading the organ. Feeling the carotid artery in the neck I noticed that the heart rate was nearly 100 per minute. I also saw that the breathing was rapid and shallow. I felt for the weak, thready radial pulse at the wrist when the State Police and ambulance arrived at the same time from two different directions. The police car followed the same ruts in the grass that the wagon had produced only moments before. As several paramedics from the ambulance ran up to the car I yelled, "Who's the crew chief?"

"I am," said a tall, blond-haired man in his 40s.

I quickly reported to the chief all vital signs, primary and secondary assessment details, and triage determinations I had made earlier. He thanked me with praise for my speedy and effective surveys, turned and yelled orders to the crew to get a backboard. He removed my mask from the man's face and attached a much more efficient one from the portable oxygen unit from the ambulance.

I asked if there was any need for further assistance and when he said "No, thank you," I moved away, packed up my gear and got back in my car.

By this time the trooper was directing traffic onto the median divider around the accident and he held it up for me to get into the traffic and continue my trip to Newtown. I remember feeling grateful that I knew both what to do and what not to do in this instance. My last thought was "Huh...the flying nuns!"

As a result of the accident that I had had several years earlier, I was on a clear multidisciplinary path. That path was emergency service and I wanted to learn as much about it as possible from every point of view. I was the Police Psychotherapist assigned to the Emergency Services Unit of Special Operations of a police department, and I had received training in negotiations and suicide prevention from the New Haven Police. In January of 1985 I took the psychodrama training part of the F.B.I. program in hostage negotiations in Washington, D.C. and returned to teach the police the F.B.I. protocols. I enjoyed working with the intelligent and capable men and women of that municipal police department and experienced many of them as extremely capable in their work and in their special assignment to hostage negotiations and to S.W.A.T. I continued to work with EMT's and even began a seminar in stress reduction and handling difficult traumatic scenes for them. By November of 1985 I was doing programs for the police, EMT's, teaching at WesConn, and seeing 25 clients per week. Things were humming along except for one small but increasingly annoying problem.

The police department had not yet paid me any part of the stipend upon which we had agreed, and I had spent almost $1500.00 to get *myself* trained in order to train them. I repeatedly spoke to the chief about this but he kept saying that it was "in process," and that I should expect to be paid soon. When I decided to complain to that city's comptroller about the slow way they were handling my funding, I was shocked to learn that he had never heard of me. He further told me that if the chief had put me on the department, he had done so "unethically and in violation of the policies of the city." I had been brought into the department, given an authorized official I.D. card and badge, used in an actual, successful scene of a barricaded, armed person, and had not done any of this with the city's blessings. I was not covered by any form of insurance. If I was injured while responding to a scene of a hostage problem, then I was not covered by any city insurance policy. I was very upset and turned over the problem to the Corporation Council of the city. When the chief heard about this charge against him he instructed his administrative officer to meet with me and arrange a "meeting of the minds" with him. I was told that there had to have been some kind of mistake and that there were funds available for me. He said that he wanted me to write up a program of training for the fall and winter of 1985 and that I would certainly get paid $1000.00 for it. In return the chief wanted me to drop all charges against him before the Corporation Council. I was willing to accept this peace agreement. By July I received a Citation from the Department officially thanking me for my "volunteered" time.

At 6:30 on Monday, August 26th we met in that town's city hall to discuss the chief's problem. I passed my badge and I.D. around to the Council members and they finally asked me what my complaint against the chief was. I said that we had worked things out and that I had no complaint. Needless to say, he was cleared of all possible wrongdoings.

I was reassigned to Special Operations and authorized a new badge with this designation. I then completed several months of training classes for the department and, despite an increasing sense that the chief no longer wanted to have me in the department, did a very successful job running a special class on the latest in interrogation techniques available at that time. I noticed that after the holidays I was no longer invited to hostage training sessions nor to any department function. I was not scheduled to teach any other classes. I began to feel like I would merely be an unused, badge-carrying part of the department. By April it was clear to me that I didn't belong in that city's police department, and I resigned. I felt quite disappointed that what had started out so potentially positive ended up on such a dark note, but by then I knew a great deal more about Emergency Services. I decided to return to my original idea to develop an organization of trainers and learners in emergency services and re-instituted the Connecticut Emergency Service Association.

I took training in Mass Disaster at the Maryland Institute for Emergency Medical Services and began public speaking on behalf of the C.E.S.A. and laying the foundations for a new and better organized recruitment program. I envisioned an organization of professionals who would be consultants to various parts of the emergency service systems of the state. The idea never even got a chance to grow beyond the formative stages. Something much more important and life-threatening took place to interrupt my planning. In the spring of 1986 I found a lump in my left testicle.

CHAPTER 11

Dr. William Hennesey sat on the stool in the examining room of his private practice and spoke frankly to me. "John, I thought before that this lump might be epididymitis, but you are right that the thickening seems to have invaded the body of the testicle itself. I think we've got testicular cancer here."

My chest constricted in a sudden rise of panic. The very word "cancer" was terrifying to me. My father had died of it in the most horrible way. "What does that come down to, Bill?" I must have had a worried expression on my face. I had been up a lot at night thinking about this recent discovery.

"It means that you should get scheduled into the hospital to perform a biopsy on the testicle. We could just perform that single operation alone, but then you'd have to have a second operation if it *was* cancerous." He tilted his head down to look at me through a different part of his field of vision. "I think we can be fairly certain that this is cancer and just remove the testicle in the original operation."

"Jesus, but the word 'cancer' scares me." I leaned back onto the white paper sheet covering the black vinyl examining table and thought this news over for a few minutes. "Bill, if I have this surgery, what will this mean about my hormone levels, and so forth? What changes could I expect?"

The physician shifted on his stool and carefully explained each of the changes that would occur. No, I would not become sterile. Yes, I would have a drop in testosterone, but it would not cause any serious changes in my muscle tone or breast tissue. Yes, it was possible to implant a prosthetic device in the empty scrotum so that the testicle would have a normal appearance. Yes, it seemed that we had caught the cancer early enough so that it would not be necessary to have any other treatment.

I remember wiping sweat off my forehead, rocking forward on the table and then nodding. "O.K., Bill. Let's go for the surgery."

"I also think we should have an oncologist in the wings in case it turns out to be something more serious."

Again, I felt a painful constriction in my chest. "I'll wait for the pathology report. I'm already feeling hysterical enough."

Over the next few weeks things moved fast. The surgery did find gross morphological changes in the tissue. The testicle was removed through an incision in the abdominal wall and a prosthetic gonad was left in its place. The pathology report confirmed a diagnosis of chorio-carcinoma mixed with eymbryonalcarcinoma.

The good news was that the malignant tumor was contained within the body of the testicle and surrounding tubules. Further good news was that these forms of cancer give off marker chemicals, beta hemato-gonadatropin and alpha feto protein. These marker chemicals allow the doctors to know whether they got all of the cancerous tissue. The bad news was that the chemical levels were quite elevated and were doubling every three days. This meant that the cancer had already spread to the lymph nodes in the abdomen. More surgery was required.

I was pretty frightened once again. It was another time for me to look into the face of death, and I was anything but accustomed. My concern was, however, not only for myself but for my family and my clients.

Isabelle, Carolyn, and I met in the living room of our home in Danbury. We began the discussion from a rational position. We addressed the possible scenarios that might occur. We tried to boost each other's morale so that we wouldn't get apprehensive about a future that was not necessarily so bright. Then we got down to feelings. We were all frightened and worried. We cried together, communally, as a family, hugged each other, and girded ourselves for the next step. I next made some contingency plans to take care of my family in the event that I was hospitalized for a long time.

With my clients I had to deal with the reality that *I* was being affected by something and that my being affected might affect them. At the time I was seeing 26 individuals or family units per week. I immediately informed all of them that they did not have to continue with me and added that I would be receiving another operation for cancer and might have to undergo chemotherapy. This latter course of treatment, I told them, would leave me rather gaunt, quite weak, and hairless. It might be a terrible thing for them to witness and might interfere with their therapy. Only one client said that he could not continue with me if I had to begin chemo, but he said that he would wait until he heard *that* news before taking a referral to another therapist from me. I felt very surprised by my clients' decisions, but I also felt wonderfully supported.

By mid-May I was talking quite a bit with my family and my mother about the upcoming surgery. One day she called me.

"Hello, son. How are you?" There was almost always a plaintive sound in my mother's voice. She often answered the phone with it as a way of putting people off that she didn't want to talk with. After talking for a while, she would drop the sound unconsciously. Usually it disturbed me, but now it seemed somehow appropriate.

"Scared, Mom." I hadn't said I was scared of anything since I was a kid. I think that I mostly wanted my mother to think that I had grown out of being frightened by things, bogeymen and such—that I had grown up—but this was different.

"I know, John...." She began to cry heavily on the phone. "Oh, John, I pray to God every day that you'll be all right. I go to mass and take communion for you. I ask God to give *me* any of your pain just to make you better." She was sobbing again.

Her words cut into me like a knife. I broke into uncontrollable crying. I felt sorry for my mother's pain. This was a familiar feeling. Also, in some far off part of myself, I felt like *I* was a parent watching my own son going through the horror of having cancer. The agony was almost more than I could stand. The parent in me was overwhelmed by my mother's and my needs.

"John, John...how could this happen to you? You were always such a good boy." I felt a sudden confusion about this statement. Was I dead in her mind? She still treated me like I was "her little boy." I shook it off.

"Mom. I don't think that goodness has anything to do with it. I am just scared. That's all. I hope things work out, but I am really afraid of the results of the surgery." Then, responding to my familiar urge to take care of her, I added, "I think everything will work out O.K., ya know?"

Her response was as empty as my attempt to soothe. "I *know that*, honey." Then she got a hold of a plan that would give her some sense of control over the situation. "Write to me son. Tell me exactly what you have to do. Share your life with me, O.K.?" Again, I had a haunted feeling about taking care of her when I was in need but I let it go.

She wanted to know everything about the procedure. She asked me to write down every detail. Whenever I had written to my mother in the past, I usually gave her very brief notes. In fact, I think I had always disliked writing to anyone, but over the next week I sat down and composed a sixpage letter describing everything that I knew about choriocarcinoma and a retroperitoneal lymph node dissection. Of course, I used words that my mother would understand. I also told her how much I loved her and what a good mother she had been to me. I didn't know why I wrote the latter, but my guess now is that I was unconsciously aware of getting close to leaving this life and I wanted to say whatever needed to be said before it was too late. Anyway, on May 22nd, while I was in a session with a client, Carolyn knocked on the office door.

I found this highly irregular and was tempted to simply say, "Not now...I'm with a client," but I asked the client if he would mind my getting the door. He said that it was O.K. with him and that he knew I would just give him the time at the end of the session. I nodded in agreement and walked over to the side of my file cabinet where I had put the entrance from the office to the house. Carolyn was standing in the doorway looking somewhat agitated. I immediately felt a shiver of fear and concern.

"What happened?" I said, thinking of Isabelle.

"I'm very sorry, John, but your mother has just died." Carolyn went on to explain briefly that my Aunt Virginia had found her sitting peacefully in her favorite armchair. The doctor at the hospital said she had died of congestive heart failure. She had been suffering attacks off and on for years but in the midst of my own fears about my mortality, I didn't realize how close she was to dying herself. I cancelled the next session. I was in total shock.

I didn't blame myself or my cancer for her death. In a way I think that she had a very peaceful departure, and I'm glad about that. But I was very concerned to know that she had received my letter. I had to discover whether she read those things I said about her being a good mother. When my brother and I went to her house to go through her belongings I found the letter on the table. As I looked at it, opened, I still needed some kind of confirmation that she had, in fact, had time to read it. One of her sisters, Virginia, then told me that she was very happy to have gotten such an outpouring of love from me. I was happy to have given it. The knowledge gave me permission to begin the mourning process for my mother.

Toward the end of May, my family and I attended Senexet House, a retreat of our Unitarian Universalist Society. It was extremely difficult for me to be there with mom's death so close behind. I kept going off by myself to cry about her...and to talk *to* her. I didn't really miss her as much as I wished that her life had been happier. Mom was an easily depressed woman and showed quite a bit of sadness on almost every visit I ever made to her. I don't know if there was any genetic or biochemical component to her persistent melancholy, but I do think that she really missed me and Dad not being around. She had been raised to think that her place was in the house and to be a wife and mother.

First, I had put an end to her motherhood by going off to college and then getting married, and then Dad ended her last attending moments as a doting wife by dying. I sometimes think that I first became a therapist to help others the way I could never seem to help my mother. Was this all there was to my being a helper? I wondered.

During the Senexet retreat one of the children broke his arm. Being an EMT I splinted, bandaged, and immobilized the fracture of the radius and ulna and drove him to the nearby hospital. I felt quite concerned for him and hovered around his tiny form as he lay, frightened, in the Emergency Room. I also assured the family that his injury was not serious and that he would probably just need to be in a cast for a while. He underwent the necessary treatment, and his family thanked me for my willingness to take care of him and deal with them despite my cancer and the death of my mother. I didn't mind.

The coffin was not the most expensive, but Ernie and I wanted it made out of wood. That was a more natural item. Metal seemed too cold for my mother's body. The oak was more warm looking than the walnut, so we chose that. We sat through the wake, like all the other wakes for members of our family, with dignity and reserve. The wake also served as an important social occasion. Many of our family seldom saw one another except at the death of a loved one. It was an odd way to meet. There was always a mixture of sadness and joy at these times as a result.

I read a eulogy over her coffin at the wake, and then we went to the burial site. Several relatives asked me if I would do their eulogies when they died. When Uncle Paul passed away one year later from cancer, I wrote and spoke *his* eulogy. It was to remind me again of the death of Mom and I cried tears for them both that year.

On June 4th, I did the first of a two-week lecture series at the Danbury Library. This particular week I spoke about the varieties and difficulties associated with human sexuality. It was very well received. The second lecture would be on "How to Do More With Your Life than Just Cope." Afterwards, a number of people came up to me and told me how inspiring I was to them. It was at this lecture that I met a man who had donated blood in my name in 1981. He asked if he could enter therapy with me, and I told him to call me for an appointment. I saw him throughout my cancer and subsequent recovery. He did quite well through his time of growth and my time of difficulty.

On Sunday, June 8th, I participated in a Mass Casualty drill of the

Monroe Emergency Medical System in Monroe, CT. We moved literally dozens of volunteer "injured" out of a school building that had "exploded" and triaged them for treatment and transport to "the hospital." It was very successful. Afterwards, in the 90-degree heat, we all went swimming with our clothes on in a portable pool the fire department had set up. It was a momentary distraction from the deep sadness I seemed to carry with me all of the time those days.

The week before I reentered the hospital was a strange one. I woke up one morning to find that a gold crown on a left rear molar was gone. I searched through the bed covers but to no avail. I must have swallowed the crown. For the next few days I sat on the toilet in the bathroom with a paper plate on a plastic plate to catch my morning stool. Then I had to focus my full attention on the dark mass of feces and mash through it with a plastic fork, looking for the missing tooth. After all, the darn thing cost several hundred dollars and I couldn't afford to simply let it go. At one point I realized the tremendous bizarreness of my life, and I just burst out laughing. For some reason the terrible had suddenly become incredibly funny. I had a plastic leg, had been diagnosed as having cancer, my mother had just died and I was sitting on the john mashing shit with a plastic fork. Could life get any more unusual? I gave up unsuccessfully after the third morning's search.

On Monday, June 16th, I entered Danbury Hospital once again. This time I was to undergo a dissection of lymph tissue from my abdomen. The radical procedure would have left me without any of those valuable "drains" for the fluid system called lymph nodes. I protested and got a compromise from my surgeon. He would do a reduced procedure in which only a little over 100 nodes would be taken out. The first day of hospitalization consisted of three enemas and several doses of laxative. They wanted the abdominal cavity to be totally quiet for the operation.

When I awoke in the hospital room I found an endotracheal tube in me. I immediately remembered a visit to my father when he was hospitalized in 1975 for exploratory abdominal surgery. It was at that time that they found him riddled with cancer of the colon. He was in a great deal of pain. He had just had the endotracheal tube removed and he had trouble talking…even swallowing. I squeezed a few tears from my eyes for my father…for myself.

The incision in my abdomen ran from under my sternum to my pubic arch. It was sore, but no where near as sore as the pains I had experienced when I was in the hospital in 1981. I felt like I would survive this much better, especially if the doctor could tell me that they had gotten all of the cancerous lymph out of me.

CHAPTER 12

The oncologist Hennesey had brought in for consultation stood at the foot of my bed. I felt a bit uncomfortable when I first met him a few days earlier, but I was beginning to like him after the four prior conversations. He was not wearing the usual smile I had seen on his face in the past. I asked him to be honest with me. Dr. Robert Cooper did not mince his words. He simply told me the news. "The b-HGB levels are still increasing. You still have cancer someplace else in your body. We have to begin chemotherapy."

"You can't do that." I pleaded. "I have been through too much already. My mother died…" I was rambling, incoherent, crying, and scared. Nothing made any sense to me. What in the name of heaven was happening? I had just turned 39. "Life begins at 40," I thought. I continued to say disconnected things.

"I've got to go down to New York City for the 4th of July celebration. I already co-rented a sailboat to anchor in the harbor. I really need to be in New York for that one." Bob Cooper was very gentle and patient with me.

"I know. I know," he said with compassion in his face. "It is terrible news to hear, but this kind of cancer—choriocarcinoma—has a very good prognosis. If we begin chemotherapy soon, you have a very good chance of being completely cured."

"…and it's now 1986 and my father died of cancer in 1976. Do you know that in '76 the Tall Ships came into the New York harbor and they had a fireworks display at the Statue of Liberty? Do you know that next week I'll be in New York harbor and watch the Tall Ships and fireworks at the Statute of Liberty? What the hell is going on, Bob?" I felt like life was just too strange. "Do you think I could just go with my wife and daughter on this one trip before I begin treatment?"

"No," he said sternly. "You could die if we don't begin therapy on Monday." The anxiety rose quickly like a shot of fire up my spine. My scalp burned. "The cancer is growing at a fantastic rate. First it enters the lymph system, then the bones, next the lungs, and finally the brain. You could be riddled with tumor cells in another week. We must begin treatment Monday."

"O.K." I said. I was becoming numb. My mind raced through a list of "things to do," and I felt like I had to prepare to die. I would call the Bengtson's and cancel my place on the boat. I had already created a contingency play with Sharon Joyce and Seab Lyon in the event that I did have to undergo more treatment. I set up a plan for them to arrange with our friends to alternately cook meals, clean, and otherwise take care of Carolyn and Isabelle if I were to stay in the hospital. I would let them know that they could start scheduling people. I wrote some checks for Carolyn to pay some of the house bills. I would have more money transferred from my savings account to checking to deal with the regular payments. I would tell my clients about beginning chemo and set up the "spread out" schedules of therapy we had discussed....

Someone had given me a book by Bernie Siegel about using visualization to fight cancer. I had never been much of a fighter in my own mind, so the idea of trying to get above the morose feeling that I was going to die *and* combat this invader inside of my body was almost completely foreign to my thinking. When I knew I was going to begin chemo, I decided to read the book and start visualizing. I read about how some people imagined that they had sharks or other wild animals in their body that were attacking and eating up the cancer cells. For me I wanted an army of soldiers. I began to visualize that I was one of a legion of warriors, on horse-back, wielding swords against the ugly black malignancy. Since one of the chemicals that I would be given was called Cis-platinum, I imagined that we were all armed with platinum swords. It seemed very noble, and I was able to maintain this visualization for an hour at a time, several times each day before the weekend passed.

On the afternoon of Monday, June 30th, the IV Team nurse found a sizeable vein in my left arm and inserted the catheter for the chemo. I would first get an injection of Bleomycin, an anti-cancer poison, followed by two other poisons administered through the IV over an eight-hour period. These were the aforementioned Cis-platinum and Vinplastin. I would also receive a chemical called Regalin which was an anti-emetic.

Its job was to reduce the desire to vomit, a common symptom of chemotherapy.

During the first six hours or so I used my visualization at least three times. I felt like this was not going to be as bad as I had feared and that I just had to ride out four months of IVs until the doctor said that I was finished with the treatment regimen.

By the end of the day the nausea began. I vomited up my supper. I vomited all over myself and projectile vomited down one side of the emesis basin and up the other onto the nurse holding it. I felt apologetic.

The nausea continued through the night. I would occasionally fall off to sleep and then awaken with a feeling of vertigo and begin retching again. By morning I realized that chemotherapy was *not* going to be *easy*!

I decided to change my visualization. I worked with the imagery until I had something that seemed to fit the job that the chemicals were doing to the cancer *and* to my body. By Tuesday evening, all three of my meals having been served on trays and removed in wash-basins, I had the new image. The army was not like a group of noble knights on horses with platinum swords. They were Huns, Goths, and Visigoths—Mongol warriors. They did not come just to fight the cancer cells. They also came to plunder and burn the villages in which the cancer cells resided. They came to destroy and maim. They were indiscriminate. I could not see them in any other form and contented myself with this imagery throughout the rest of my treatments.

I watched the fireworks at the Statue of Liberty on television from my hospital bed. I remembered 1976 and could not understand the coincidence of my father having cancer then and my having it in 1986 when the Tall Ships returned to New York Harbor. It was eerie.

After the first week of steady IV drip was over, I remained in the hospital for several more days to regain some strength. I had begun to lose weight and felt quite weak from the lack of sleep and the persistent regurgitating.

I began seeing my clients the day I returned home. I checked in with each one of them at the end of each session to see how that person or couple or family felt about my weakened state. Almost all of them reported that they did not notice any difference with my focus or ability to facilitate them in their process. That was all that mattered. Kendall, the one client who felt uncomfortable with what I might look like in another month decided to terminate. I offered to refer him to a colleague, but he said he felt like he wanted to "go it" on his own. I continued my work with the other 20 plus clients.

At mealtime I was able to eat soup, especially chicken noodle soup, and a few other light foods. Meats and rough vegetables were out of the question. I could neither keep them down nor even look at them without having a gagging reflex. After two weeks home I could eat a few more complex foods, but it was time for me to return to the hospital. I decided to bring a guitar with me to distract me during the long hours. I bought an inexpensive solid-body guitar and small amplifier with earphones so I could play without disturbing the other patients. I was ready to return.

The second course of treatment was designed to be the worst. Bob had warned me about this ahead of time. The doses would all be increased, and I would have even more nausea and vertigo than before. At the end of the first day, my head was swimming and my throat was sore from all of the vomiting. The Regalin was also having some kind of affect on my body. I was feeling agitated and kept trying to get out of bed and walk around to "work off" the nervousness. I grew short-tempered with visitors and often asked them to leave after only a five- or 10-minute visit.

At night, if I slept, I would have the weirdest dreams. They were usually about worms or shit or eating foul things (a theme of disgust and nausea, I guess).

Despite my exercising and visualizing, I began to get depressed and more concerned with death. I also felt a certain despair, as if my God had abandoned me. I felt incredibly alone in my fear and abandonment. I felt pretty hopeless after two more days of constant retching. The Regalin was also making me quite nervous. I called for a psychiatric consultation.

The psychiatrist, wearing a white lab coat, sat at the foot of my bed with a clipboard on his knees. I knew him from having worked with him on a client of mine whom he had hospitalized for me and from having lunch with him on another occasion.

"So...what would you say your general mood was these days?"

"Um...frightened...sad...and worried about a lot of religious and philosophical things...like what my life is all about and why a God would even allow these horrible things to happen to me...and," I added, "...tired of throwing up...but that's not a feeling."

"Un huh...and do you feel like anyone here at the hospital is against you?"

"What? Matt, if you mean 'am I paranoid?', the answer is 'no'."

"Do you think that you have any control over other people or that you can make people do things with your mind?"

Recognizing the questions of a familiar intake procedure I said, "Matt, I can save you a lot of time here. I am oriented in the usual spheres. My mood is anxious and depressed. I have no auditory, visual, gustatory, kinesthetic or olfactory hallucinations. I do not think that people are talking about me behind my back or that people want to get me. I have some difficulty concentrating and paying attention which may be soft signs of my depression or due to chemotherapy. I do not have any difficulty managing my daily living activities except when I'm throwing up and mostly, I called for you because I'm afraid that I'm going to die and I need some help with this feeling."

He nodded thoughtfully throughout this narrative and then persisted in a totally mechanical tone. "Do you have any feelings that you want to do any harm to yourself or to anyone else?"

"Matt, for Christ sake…talk to me. Stop using the goddamn Mental Status Exam to put distance between us. I'm frustrated here and you are not helping."

He nodded.

"Look…I have no suicidal or homicidal ideations. Furthermore, my memories seem unimpaired and I don't have any compulsive behaviors that I can't stop. I do have obsessive thoughts about my possible death and the meaning of my life, O.K.?"

"Do you feel like I'm persecuting you now?"

"Matt. I feel like you are being an inappropriate 'professional' when what I need is to talk about my fear of dying from cancer. I feel like I urgently need to deal with a whole bunch of existential issues."

"Well. I think I can make a schedule with you and we could begin to talk about your fears." He was totally aloof. I was trying to reach out to another human being for some support and all I was facing was a professional role. He *was* the *role* called psychiatrist.

"Have you ever had a serious illness where you thought you'd die?" I needed to hear if he understood what I was going through.

"Why do you ask?" He was working to fend off any closeness or intimacy.

"You aren't going to answer my questions, are you?"

"I don't think I'm here to discuss myself." He was doing the role to the nth degree. "I think that I can see you…." He flipped the pages of his appointment book. "…on Friday at 2 p.m. O.K.?"

"No. It's not O.K., Matt. I really just want to express a few of my fears to you and I really wish you didn't feel it was so necessary to 'act' like the 'doctor' with me right now." I was pleading for his humanity.

Rising from the chair he said in a controlled tone, "Well, I'll be back on Friday and we can talk then." He walked briskly from the room without so much as a "goodbye."

The nightmares were very disturbing to me. I often awoke sweating and then began to vomit or have dry heaves. In one of my dreams I was about to get on a plane and leave everyone else behind. I didn't want to get aboard, but it seemed like that was what I had to do. The vision of the plane frightened me. The therapist in me told me it was my fear of dying.

On Thursday I had another visit from a woman who had attended my lecture series at the Danbury Library. She would come into my room and begin talking *at* me. She seldom heard my responses and sometimes didn't seem to hear anything I asked her. After a while I gave up trying to have any meaningful contact and just lay back on the pillow. Even though I was getting bored with her visit, I began to feel a great deal of unusual agitation. I started to focus on this sensation when I felt my right hand tightening. I looked down at the contorted fingers and felt the muscles of my back begin to constrict. Something different was happening to me. Was I actually going crazy or was this something physical?

When my left hand contracted and my mouth began to pull back into an involuntary grin I realized what was occurring. I tried to get the visitor's attention. She did not hear my pleas for assistance. I spoke up. She spoke on. Finally in anger I yelled, "Damn it! Would you get the nurse?"

"Is it something *I* said?" she inquired. "I really didn't mean to upset you, Dr. Gagnon. Why, I really only was saying that when I got the flowers on Wednesday...well...I didn't know who had sent them and...."

I managed to wrap my distorted claw around the white shaft with the red button on it and press down. She was caught in mid sentence.

"...and he said he knew that I *loved* geraniums...."

The nurse came rushing into the room. She looked at my rapidly tightening face. "I'm going into tetany...." She hesitated. "Clonus...clonic seizure...whatcha call it," I added through clenched teeth. I was biting at the words.

The visitor seemed to regain her composure and tried to begin again. I cut her off. "Just leave, please."

"Well. I certainly didn't mean to upset you."

My jaw was very tight. "It's not you. I'm sick."

She waved a hand in understanding as she backed into Bob and two nurses who were rushing into the room.

"My, my, my," Bob said with a broad smile on his face. "Will you look at that." He was pointing to my twisted smile. "*Rictus sardonicus*," he explained to the nurse.

"Thank you, doctor, for the explanation. Now, will you get me out of this?" I was really smiling in my heart at his need to use me as a classic example of clonus and my face was already pulled into an involuntary and unnatural grin. It was an appropriate congruity.

The nurse rushed out of the room to get the Benadryl and another medication while Bob just looked at me, smiled and shook his head. "Will you look at that. It's...."

"...dystonia!" I was barely able to say the word.

"Very good!" Bob raised his eyebrows. "How'd you know that? Very good." His voice mimicked in inflection the posture of the eyebrows. He shook his head at me and laughed.

The nurse came back with the medications and within an hour the seizure had passed. I was taken off of Regalin and placed on another anti-emetic. The vomiting increased and so did my nightmares and day fears.

On Friday at about 2:00 p.m., a nurse came into the room while I was playing my guitar to myself.

"Hi there. I've got a Bleomycin injection for you."

"O.K." I stopped playing.

"No...please don't stop. It sounds nice."

"You can't hear much without an amplifier but...O.K." I started playing some chords and soon found a song that I could play and sing while she sat on the edge of the bed and held the needle and slowly injected the medication into the IV tubing that snaked into a deep vein in the bicep of my right arm. Bleo was a potentially damaging chemical and had to be injected over a timed period. In undiluted concentrations it would actually destroy some of the tissue along the inside wall of the vein. I would just have to wait until the plunger was all the way down. I played on.

"Oh." Matt said as he walked into the room.

"Hi, Matt, I'll be finished in...how long?"

She looked at her watch. "Another two minutes."

He turned on the spot and left the room. I felt uncomfortable with his exit and wondered if he would wait the two minutes before coming back.

When the nurse left I got up, put on a robe and took my noisily whirring auto infusion pump on wheels for a walk to the nurses' station. The IV line hung from beneath the robe and the bags of chemo swung back and forth on the hanger above the pump.

At the station the nurse told me that the psychiatrist had walked out of my room and without hesitation had gone to see another patient in another part of the hospital. I felt irritated by his not sticking around for two lousy minutes. Something about this situation felt awfully familiar to me. I was aching to get on with the process of talking about fear, and the way I was being ignored was all too reminiscent of my prior hospitalization and the way that people were unable or refused to deal the feeling of anger.

I called up the operator and asked for him to be paged. When I got his voice on the telephone I asked him when he would come to see me.

"Well, obviously you are doing just fine and are not in any clinical crisis so...let me see....I could see you this coming Monday."

"That is unsatisfactory with me," I replied in an upset voice. "I have nightmares every night, seldom get any sleep because I am afraid of these nightmares and worry about death during the day when I'm awake. I really would just like to have a half hour of your time today."

"No can do," he said in a matter of fact tone. "I don't really think you are feeling *that* badly."

I thought to myself, "How the fuck does he know what I feel? It's not easy for me to admit that I'm totally terrified and I have taken that risk with my psych consult only to be told that I'm not 'feeling that badly'!" I replied, "Matt, you are no longer on my case."

"Huh!" he asked without seeming to understand.

"You are fired!" I slammed down the receiver.

Later that day I called a colleague and prior supervisor of mine, George Steinfeld, and arranged for him to come to see me at the hospital on a professional basis. He agreed.

George helped me to face the possibility of my death. He even gave me a tape that had a guided visualization on it about letting go and welcoming death. I found it a bit disturbing and didn't use it, but I did find George's visits helpful. Psychiatry also sent me another consultant. His name was Brian Quigley, a very English sort who was quite easy to be with and seemed to enjoy spending time with me talking about his prior experiences. He also reduced some concern I had about suddenly being placed on Thorazine. I knew that this medication was only for psychotic patients, and I wondered if the prior consultant had decided that I was psychotic. Dr. Quigley informed me that it was also a very powerful antiemetic (he described another story from his past about how a woman on a sheep farm somewhere had been helped with this medication) and concluded by reiterating that I was on a small subclinical dose of the medication to alleviate the nausea. He was quite right; it did help. I found that within a few days, the vomiting had subsided quite a bit. I was glad about this and secretly wished that it would vanish altogether, but the improvement was greatly appreciated.

I always enjoyed his visits because of the distraction he created by his stories. I was never aware of his trying any type of therapeutic intervention with me, however. Maybe his "story telling" was the therapeutic intervention he made. I don't know. I do know that I enjoyed his company and his pleasant demeanor.

The most helpful therapist I met during the entire ordeal was not even a therapist. It was Bob Cooper. He shared with me fears he himself had had when he was once hospitalized for surgery. I felt an empathy and concern from him that was very welcome. He told me that I was very brave to deal with the constant feeling of vertigo that I had. I didn't understand. He told me that it was far worse than the physical pain that I had had in the previous hospitalization in '81. To illustrate this he said, "If you are fighting an army and you wound some of the soldiers, those who are wounded, if not mortally so, will still be able to fight a while longer. If, however, you make them nauseous with vertigo, they will immediately be struck to their knees and be unable to go on." This added a certain noble meaning to the nausea that I *had* to feel in order to get well, and I was inspired by his words to face it more bravely. Notice, I said "to get well." With George's, possibly Brian's and especially Bob's help I no longer thought that I was going to die. I wasn't sure about some of the other patients on the ward, however, and my concern for myself shifted to others that I encountered each day.

There was one patient who had already lost his hair. He was completely bald and I would see him walking, gaunt and hollow-eyed down the hall. He stared ahead like a zombie, like the walking dead. He looked quite disturbed, and I was never able to get a coherent response from him. I wondered what would happen to him. He looked so sick, so doomed.

Another patient was a roommate of mine. He seemed well enough. He had lost his hair but was not so skinny and he had an artificially buoyant spirit that covered his own impending death. He was a model airplane store owner and also raised show dogs. He taught me quite a bit about how to select a dog as a pet. One day he told me, with a sudden catch in his voice, that he knew he was going to die. I was shocked by the news. I did not want him to die. I asked him how he could be so certain and he said that the doctors had given up on trying to beat his cancer and had removed him from all treatment. He was in the hospital to die. I felt a cold horror at this idea. He asked for a single room—he wanted to be alone. I never saw him again.

My new roommate was a young man who was very religious. He was a Baptist and continually read religious books and the Bible. He often talked to me about his "personal relationship with Jesus" and how he was "saved." I told him that I was still quite confused about my own religious beliefs but that I was willing to talk with him about his. He told me that if I gave myself to Jesus as my personal savior that I would be saved from death by eternal life. This sounded something like the messages that I had received in Catholicism as a child but without the associated guilt.

When he saw my guitar he told me that he would trade something with me. He would play me a song about Jesus if I would play him a song that I enjoyed. He picked up my instrument and carefully figured the three chords that he would play. The sound was quite thin. The guitar had no sounding box behind it but when he had the three chords figured out he began.

"Jesus loves me..." the song began. He sang it like an innocent child.

His voice was as thin as the sound of the guitar behind it. The tune was extremely simple and the words even simpler, but after a few verses a soft welling began in my chest. The passion was incredible. I felt a powerful sense of LOVE. I spell it with capitals because it was undirected. I didn't just love an object, someone. I felt totally loved and in love with all life. It was a strange new feeling for me. My therapist mind questioned if this was some kind of delusional feeling, but after a while I just gave in to it. I looked at this young man and I felt love for him. I cared what would happen to him and I cared that others on the ward would recover.

When he finished and smiled benevolently on me, I felt a little embarrassed and had some difficulty admitting to him the reaction I had had to his song—to the innocent and yet inspirational quality of it. He looked at me and said "God loves you, you know." I abruptly burst into tears and was struck by the suddenness. I couldn't stop crying and I realized that he had said something that I had ached to hear for a long time. It was quite a while before I was able to recover my composure and remember that I was supposed to play a song for him. He listened with pleasure as I sang. I don't remember what it was. I do remember that I kept thinking of how ugly my own ornate song was compared with the simplicity and beauty of his.

He was moved to another hospital as his lymphoma grew. He became more and more ill, and within a few months he died. I don't know if he died peacefully, knowing that God or Jesus was with him, but I do know that I missed him and his simple religious and existential views. He made an impact on me that I shall never forget.

After my second treatment I had to remain in the hospital for another week just to get over the devastating effects that the chemo had had on me. I was now losing hair and was able to run my fingers over my scalp and come away with clumps of the brown locks in my hands. My eyes looked sunken and I had dropped in weight to about 170 pounds. Bob Cooper placed me on hyperalmentation, a kind of IV food, and I also underwent an operation to have a special "port" placed in my chest to receive future IVs. My veins had suffered, and I had red streaks down both arms showing the paths of the damaged, irritated vessels beneath my skin. I had to reschedule all of my clients to the following week. They didn't seem to mind.

When I got back to work, several clients were surprised at my appearance, but I strove to keep my focus on their issues and to work as clearly as possible with them. They seemed to profit from my interpretations and interventions and neither I nor they felt that I was in any way adversely affected by my own condition. In fact, several of them remarked that I had become "different" since being in the hospital and they felt more comfortable with me—that I was "more human" than before. Was this an unexpected benefit of having been so sick, so near death again? I thought, "Maybe I'll find that suffering can be a beneficial form of personal growth." I then realized I wouldn't recommend it to anyone, that's all. I worked on keeping my personal musings to myself.

Sandy was a woman in her early forties. She was a senior supervisor for the telephone company and had come to therapy to learn "how to be more assertive" with her boss and coworkers, particularly a younger woman by the name of Tammy. Tammy had just been hired to work switchboard. She was a college student hired for the summer but from the way Sandy described her, she was a "brat...who seemed to be getting her first period."

In a previous session, Sandy had imagined confronting Tammy and had done so only with a great deal of prodding and coaching from me. I was exceedingly exhausted after that particular session. This day, despite my red veins, gaunt face and the fact that I had just finished seeing five clients, I felt eager to pick up with Sandy where we had left off last time.

She entered the office wearing a flowered blouse with a light green skirt. The combination was attractive and yet appropriately comfortable for her work setting. Sandy hesitated at the doorway, gave me a broad smile and said, "You look well today!"

I furrowed my brow in bewilderment and questioned, "I do?"

"Yes, despite all that you've been through, John, you seem...well...you seem...I don't know...somehow calm and peaceful. In fact, you look healthy!"

I didn't feel calm and peaceful, I felt nauseous.

Sandy stepped over to the couch and sat lightly on the front edge. She nodded as if to say, "There!"

I took my place in my favorite firm chair, turned it to face the couch, noticed that the curtain on the artificial window behind her head was wrinkled and then leaned forward on my elbows to start the session.

"I don't feel well, Sandy, but maybe I look better than I feel."

She smiled in an artificial way so that her eyes squinted and nodded again.

I began to wonder whether she was projecting her own well feelings onto me or was so out of contact that she wasn't really seeing me at all. She interrupted my reverie by dropping back against the couch.

"I've been doing a lot of thinking since our last session and I realize that I never did finish the anger which I felt for Tammy and the bratty way that she refuses to take breaks when I tell her. She is a workaholic. It's like she just...wants to run the whole show. She's such an immature child." She hit the seat next to her as she said this.

"You want to hit Tammy?" I said jokingly while gesturing toward Sandy's fisted hand.

"No...I'm just so darn pissed at her for ignoring me."

I don't know why, but I suddenly began to remember an earlier session in which we had done some grief work on Sandy's daughter, Estelle, who was killed by a school bus driver. He, apparently, had failed to wait for her to pass safely in front of the bus and cross the street to her home. The daughter was killed instantly. Sandy had kept a lot of her sad feeling bottled up inside of her until I had her visualize that scene in her mind. As she thought of the bus striking Estelle, Sandy had done a considerable amount of crying and ended the session by saying, "That's over now." I remember that I didn't believe her. I decided to share my thought.

"I don't understand why, but when you talked about being ignored I thought of Estelle. Did Estelle tend to ignore you?"

Sandy looked surprised. "That's weird. I was just thinking about Estelle too. No. Estelle always listened to me...but...I was remembering sitting in the police car being driven to the hospital. I kept believing that Estelle was alive—that somehow she had survived the accident. I asked the officer, but he just said, 'We'll find out what happened when we reach the E.R.'"

"So, he ignored you and wouldn't tell you what you wanted to know."

She visibly slumped down in her seat and began to tremble. "None of them would tell me. I begged the doctor and the nurse...and the ward secretary, but they kept saying that they couldn't tell me anything until my husband arrived."

"You must have thought that Estelle was dead or at least very ill, no?"

"I was positive that she was dead but they wouldn't tell me for sure." Sandy's shoulders slumped even more.

"Sandy," I said as I rose from my chair, teetering to one side from the sudden drop in my blood pressure, "if this was the emergency room of the hospital where would you be? Where would the doctor, nurse and ward secretary be? Place them by arranging the chairs."

Sandy proceeded to move some of my furniture, pointing to and fro until she had located herself in front of my desk (now being used as the E.R. ward's counter behind which sat the secretary). Sandy said that she imagined the doctor and the nurse behind her and standing between her and the couch, which would serve as "the curtained cubicle in which Estelle lay." When Sandy was finished, she sat down in front of the "secretary", and began to relive the scene.

"They have..."

"*You* have," I interrupted.

"You have no right to ignore my requests about my daughter!" Sandy then looked up at me with pleading eyes and added, "They ignored my request to see her body!"

"Tell them that." I gestured to the "secretary chair" and also to the "doctor and nurse" position.

Spinning around in her seat, Sandy turned bright red in the face as she blurted out, "You can't ignore a mother's need to see her baby. My baby was in an accident. Why can't I see her?" Sandy was screaming now. "I know she's dead and I want to see her body!"

"They won't let you see her and they won't tell you that she's dead."

"You fucking bastards....I hate you all."

"Yes."

"I hate you all. You are supposed to be trained professionals. You know best how to deal with a mother who has lost her child. Who the hell do you think you are and why do you keep ignoring me?" Sandy now struck her leg with her fist.

"Don't hit yourself, Sandy." I put a pile of cushions on another chair next to hers. "Hit this instead," I said.

"You rotten, rotten people. You have no right to keep me from knowing. Stop ignoring me. Stop it, stop it, stop it." Sandy pounded on the cushions until her anger was vented. She then collapsed into sobbing.

I carefully approached her and asked, "May I touch you?"

She nodded and I placed one hand on her shoulder. The sobbing increased with this support.

"I never got to see my baby. I was later told that she was dead when Charles [her husband] arrived, but I never saw Estelle. I wanted to hold her and to tell her 'goodbye'."

"O.K., Sandy. Go through the curtains to the stretcher where Estelle is lying. Hold her and talk to her." The couch had a large flowered throw pillow on it. I hoped that Sandy's visualization would allow her to make that pillow into Estelle.

Sandy slowly rose from the seat in front of my desk and crossed the room toward the couch. A small black chair stood between her and the couch. She kicked it to one side saying, "Get the fuck out of my way, *doctor*."

Sandy gently knelt in front of the sofa and leaned over and wrapped her arms around my large throw pillow. She spoke softly and lovingly. "Estelle, my baby, my baby....'" She cried for a long time and then spoke again, "I love you so much, but you had to die. You were brain damaged by the accident. You would have been a vegetable if you had lived." She stroked the cushion as if caressing the hair of her daughter.

"So, you know that it is better that she died and that you have to suffer her death?"

"Yes! That's right! It *is* better! I release you, Estelle. I love you and I release you to die." With this, Sandy let go of the pillow, slumped to the floor and completed her grief. When she finally looked up at me sitting on the floor next to her she said, "God…your arms are all marked up and you look so pale. Are you o.k.?"

"Don't worry about me right now, Sandy. You just let your baby die. You've been denying the rest of this grief because you had something else in the way."

"Was it my anger at the hospital staff?"

"Yep. They ignored you and it was Tammy's ignoring you that got you in touch with this deeper frustration, this earlier memory."

"Oh my God!"

"Oh my God, what?"

"If Estelle had lived, she'd be exactly Tammy's age now. Dear Lord, but that's incredible."

"I never cease to be amazed at how the mind works, Sandy."

After a quick look at her watch she added, "Should I try to confront Tammy right now?"

"I think we can save working on how to deal with Tammy's rebellion until another session. You've done plenty today."

"Un huh…yeah, I have!" Sandy smiled in a genuine way this time.

By the time I reentered Danbury Hospital for the next ordeal of treatments I had lost all of my hair and was reduced to drinking only broth or jello. I would usually vomit the jello. At the hospital I received chemo *and* IV nutrients constantly. One day I decided to try an ice cream soda. I had a growing desire to eat substantial food again. This was a good sign. I finished the chocolate drink and actually enjoyed the taste, but before I could call the nurse to tell her the good news I puked the entire thing all over the covers and the floor of the room. I was quite embarrassed and gave up trying to keep anything down.

Water by itself was all I took by mouth. The hyperalmentation would be my only food for now. My weight continued to descend to 150 pounds. In the mirror I reminded myself of a victim of Auschwitz. My mustache was gone as well, and I looked like a shell of my former self. I had to go on, however; I was now determined that I would defeat the cancer successfully and become well again. There was still much more for me to do before I died.

CHAPTER 13

On August 20th, 1986, I came home. On the 21st I worked 14 client-hours. One of these sessions was with the Brown family. Actually it consisted of the father, mother, daughter, son, and the daughter's sixteen-year-old boyfriend, Ron. The age of the boyfriend would be unimportant except that the daughter was twenty-one and was still living at home with no apparent plans for her future. She was quite bright but was, in many ways, emotionally like a late teenager herself. The parents were quite worried, and they often thought that they should intervene and just "stop Nancy's nonsense" and "get her off to college where she belonged."

I had been working with this family since before my cancer, and they were rapidly approaching an important piece of insight. In one session I had used family sculpture to observe how an individual member of the system viewed the relationship of all members to one another. This is a process where a person is permitted to tell everyone present where to sit or what posture (like a statue) to take in relation to every other person. This sculptured metaphor is quite descriptive and informative. Each one had his or her own version of the arrangement of people in the Brown family sculpture (including, of course, the extended member, Ron) but all of them had one item in common. Nancy was always placed in the exact middle of the arrangement. What stability was Nancy facilitating by her idiosyncratic behavior? What function was she serving in this family? How was she central? I intended to find out.

I saw the concern in their eyes when they saw me totally hairless and baby-faced. "Hello, fabily," I said like a child with adenoids. "Hi Ron." The ice was broken. Several laughed.

Everyone nodded or murmured, "Hi, John." We spent a few moments discussing how each person felt about my appearance, and then I went into my usual warmup.

"Before beginning the actual work of today's session, as always, let's check in with everyone to see how they are." Turning in the father's direction I opened the door. "Ted?..."

When each had said how he or she was feeling or what that person was expecting out of the session that day, I offered the following exercise.

"How about we return to doing the sculptures this week in order to find out more about their meaning?" I looked around the small group and saw them nodding approval. "What I'm thinking is that I'd like each of you to do a sculpture of how the family would look if we removed Nancy and Ron from the picture, if she went off and got married, for example." The father winced, looked down at the floor, and nodded.

"Ted. How'd you like to start off this time?"

The father looked up. His face looked sheepish and innocent. "Me? Uh...O.K....sure." He got up uneasily and began to direct each member of the group into a position. He attempted to bring Nancy into the center but then he remembered that she and Ron were out of the sculpture. He looked terribly perplexed. Finally, after ten minutes of various permutations of arrangement, he settled on the following placement. Mother (Alice) was on one side of the room with the son, Bobby. Since the client for the next session had not yet arrived, Ron and Nancy were put out in the waiting room. Ted stood alone behind my desk at the opposite end of the room from Alice and Bobby. He was facing away from them as well.

"Well. This is an interesting arrangement." I leaned on my cane as I hobbled between the three separated members of the family. "So, for you, Ted, when Nancy and Ron are not here, you and Alice are separated?"

Ted looked dismal but nodded in agreement. "That's all I could seem to come up with."

Next, Alice did her sculpture. While the exact distances were not the same, the overall gestalt or configuration was.

For Bobby, Mom and Dad held each other's hands and looked into each other's eyes. He was standing on either side of them with his hand on each shoulder.

"Bobby. You look like you are trying to keep them from moving apart?"

"Yes. I don't want them to stand apart. I want them to love each other."

"So, if Nancy goes off then you would have to hold mom and dad together?"

"I don't want you to do that, Bobby," Alice said. "We have been leaning on Nancy long enough. I think it's time for us to talk, Ted."

He looked at the floor and dropped her hands. "Yes, it is. We've kept Nancy our baby. I know that I've wanted her never to grow up. I don't know what's happened to *us*, Alice, but I feel like I don't even know who you are." They backed up and stared at one another like they were seeing each other for the first time.

In subsequent sessions I attempted to investigate the possibility that they had buried their affection for one another and had replaced it with an infantilizing love for Nancy. As the sessions proceeded, however, it became more and more evident that Nancy was the only glue that had kept them from divorcing years before. They concluded the therapy with divorce counseling and both parted as amicable and wise friends.

While, in my heart, I had hoped that my hypotheses about them and the necessity of Nancy as a stabilizing influence in their marriage were wrong, I was able to stand back and let the natural process of divorce occur. I was proud of myself. They were happy about the outcome. Nancy and Ron later split up. Nancy did decide, of her own volition, to go to college, and Ron was content to go to trade school to learn to be an auto mechanic, something he had always wanted to do. Occasionally I hear from Alice telling me how Nancy and Bobby are doing.

"Bob, what's with the tremendous difficulty I always seem to have breathing?" I was sitting on the edge of the hospital bed in the cancer ward awaiting my Bleomycin shot which started the fever that announced the beginning of the nauseating treatment process.

"Well, it's too early to tell, but it might be a little bit of pulmonary fibrosis. Bleomycin tends to either cause fevers or produce some minor lung damage. Like the brown stripes you have on your skin from the other chemicals, some of the damage is reversible." He smiled at me. "Let's focus our energy on getting this cancer right now. All of your chemical markers are negative. That means that as of now the cancer is dead. We still need to do this last part of the regimen, however, to give you the highest probability of permanent recovery."

With a temperature of 103, I gave myself over to the last week of vomiting and dizziness. My hopes were high.

I had to undergo two days of hyperalmentation following the end of treatment and was released from the hospital on September 16th. I immediately started seeing my clients. There were seven clients on Wednesday, eight on Thursday, and the remainder on Friday. On Friday I received a call from my brother.

He told me that our mother's estate was going to probate and that we had some initial lawyers fees to deal with. He took care of them from an advance account which was released by the attorney from my mother's bank savings, a few thousand dollars. Just the thought of negotiating money after Mom's death made me sad again. It would have been fine with me if she had spent every last nickel before she died. I thought again of her tendency not to go out or to spend money on herself. I felt sorry for the difficult life she had. I certainly did not look forward to the eventual job of dividing up the property and the sale of the house in Derby. In the last few months before she died, she had only left the house by ambulance to go to the hospital whenever she had great difficulty breathing.

Saturday I spent most of my time in bed. I felt exceedingly tired. The week had been quite taxing, and I was still having trouble getting enough air to do simple jobs like walking across a room. My doctor told me that weakness was a natural outcome of chemo but that it would eventually pass as I got back to eating regular foods again. I was still unable to keep down most meats, but any pasta dish was both delicious and digestible.

Since I was still vomiting several times during the day and night, I tried to sleep on the couch Saturday night. I lay in the living room and looked back over the past four months of agony. I was glad that it was over. I would get stronger now. As I thought about this, my breath became more and more constricted. At first I thought it might be a minor anxiety attack, but I was not feeling anxious.

I sat up on the edge of the bed and tried to catch my breath. I was huffing and wheezing like a runner who had just finished a 100 meter run. The feeling of not having enough air got worse.

A little after 1:00 a.m. I was having accompanying chest pain, mostly on the left side. The thought of a heart attack occurred to me, but my doctor had said that my heart was very strong, and I realized that I was probably having a bout with the pulmonary disease brought on by the chemo. I called for an ambulance.

After being treated with oxygen and steroids, Bob Cooper placed me on a strong regimen of prednisone. I was right in my suspicions. I had pulmonary fibrosis. The function tests and X-rays showed that I was getting only about two thirds of the oxygen that most people got. Walking up a flight of stairs became a tremendous difficulty for me, and I felt like I was 90 years old. In addition to this, my ears began to ring. Another possible side effect of the treatment was tinnitus. It was the result of damage to the eighth cranial nerve, the one that conducts impulses from the ear to the brain. I would always hear everything through a high-pitched ringing from that day forward. I became discouraged.

The third side effect was Raynaud's disease. The blood vessels in my hands and foot would now constrict unexpectedly. My fingers became white and sometimes numb without warning. This would not have been a problem in the summer, but it was now fall and the weather was getting colder and colder. I always wore a hat on my nearly bald head and gloves on my hands. Sometimes I would soak my hands in warm water between sessions with clients. I still have Raynaud's disease, but it has decreased in intensity.

When services at the Unitarian Universalist Society of West Redding started up again in the fall, I began attending. At the first meeting of the Society members were welcomed back after the summer. We have always had a tradition at our church. It is called Milestones, and it consists of a time when members of the congregation can stand up and tell something about a success or tragedy that has recently occurred in their lives and receive the applause or consolation of the rest of the membership. During this day's Milestone sharing I stood up. I looked pale and thin in my clothing. My hair was barely visible on my head. I was going to announce the obvious, that I had successfully been treated for cancer and that I was returning to my life once again. Instead all I said was, "Contrary to popular belief, I did not spend the summer in a Hari Krishna cult." Somehow the laughter was a relief to the tension I felt and anyone that counted in my life already knew the triumph that overcoming cancer had been for me. It wasn't necessary to say any more than that. I sat down to the applause and tears of my loving community of friends.

I also signed up for the special adult program that was being offered at the Society on the reading and study of a new book that had been published by a local psychiatrist. The book, *The Road Less Traveled* by M. Scott Peck of New Milford, was a best-seller, and a number of us were interested in examining his perspective on leading a more healthy life. I was also still searching for some kind of meaning to all the pain and suffering I continually had to go through, despite the way I had dedicated my life to helping others. It didn't seem to make any sense to me at one level—as if I were dealing with life from an "exchange mentality." I expected to get what I gave. At another level, however, I realized that bad things happened to lots of people and that it would be grandiose to think that life would single me out for suffering. Nevertheless, my friends persisted in thinking of me as a "modern-day Job" and often asked me how I could deal with all my trials. I usually mumbled something about not knowing how I could and being perfectly honest about how worried I was by my illnesses. I also worried about what the next bad thing would be.

In the workshop on Peck's book I rethought my attitudes and perceptions about cancer. I would have done as much for any client of mine, but it was different when I was the one with the problems. One of the most important aspects of the Friday night sessions was the support of my friends. At one point Carolyn Holt gave me a gold-colored medal on a blue ribbon saying that I was "a champion for having come through my difficulties of the past several years." I began to think about people and about heroism. It seemed to me that it was fairly easy to win a battle ribbon for doing what was expected of one during war-time, but that people are not recognized for the way they persist in the face of life's daily vicissitudes. I had always felt a profound respect and admiration for my clients and others who had to face suffering in their lives. They were heros in the truest sense of the word even though society would seldom recognize or honor them as such. I thought of Copeland's musical composition, "Fanfare for the Common Man." Common people deserve fanfares for their bravery. I was not accustomed to thinking of myself as one of the brave ones, however.

The adult course proceeded quite well. I learned many things from Peck. One of the ones that stands out in my mind is that "love is not a feeling." It is, for him, an act of "doing." In other words, if I do something for someone when I want to do it—because it pleases me—then I am not necessarily doing something loving for them. If, on the other hand, I don't feel like doing something kind or caring for another but I do it anyway, then this is a real loving act. I didn't totally agree with Peck's apparent suggestion that one doesn't *feel love* when doing the unpleasant task for the loved one, but it gave me something to think about. I realized that I was truly loved by so many people who had done small things for me throughout my illness, and I realized that, when I was feeling quite ill and was still seeing my clients, that I was showing them a great deal of love. I felt good about this. I liked my loving behavior and that of my friends. I have always believed that by accepting a place in the world that one takes on a necessary responsibility for the life of others as well as oneself. This statement of Peck's was an affirmation to that belief.

On December 16th, 1986 I was at midlife—40 years old. Funny...I didn't feel like I was half way through my existence on this planet. I certainly didn't feel "over the hill" (a popular insult inscribed on assorted coffee mugs, T-shirts, hats, etc. for persons who hit this socially significant birthday). I had been mostly happy to be over the cancer and to be recovering. I had expected a party of some kind but exactly what, I wasn't sure.

Steve was not a friend with whom I got together very often, so when he called I felt confused by the urgency with which he said, "I would really like to get together with you and for you to come over to the house for a while right now...uh...and I will need a lift back to your house later because Jeanne has the car and will pick me up there. O.K.?"

"O.K., Steve," I said in a puzzled way. "You want to get together 'for a while'?"

"Uh...yes. I *really* would like to see you right now and I'll need a lift back to your house to get a ride from Jeannie." He said this with much more conviction and self-assurance. I was still confused by the whole thing but decided that I was just missing something. However....

It was my birthday. This had to be a ruse to get me out of the house. I would go along. "O.K., then. I'll be over in about 15 minutes. Honey," I called in to Carolyn in the kitchen. "I'm going over to Steve Clidas' for a while. I'll be back later." I smiled but she didn't seem to notice.

"All right, John. Have a good time." She came up on her toes as she gave me a kiss and then turned back to the dishes at the sink.

On the drive over to Steve's I wondered exactly what Carolyn had in mind. Obviously it was going to be a party and there would be some of my friends there. I contemplated exactly who she might invite. I must have come up with about a dozen of my best friends.

Steve acted very strange throughout my visit and we chatted about all kinds of things: my psychotherapy practice, the reduction in my nausea and the growth of approximately 1/4 inch of straight, brown hair, his students at school and his new practice in massage therapy. At about 5:30 p.m., Steve said that he needed that ride and emphasized again that he would meet his wife at my place. I drove him back and was a little disappointed to find no unusual cars in the driveway. Maybe this was *not* a ruse. Maybe I had read the whole thing wrong and Carolyn was going to have a quiet, family dinner for me.

As I stepped across the front portal I was immediately greeted by Carolyn who grabbed me and gave me a great big kiss. Equally as sudden, the entire house seemed to burst forth with the peal, "Happy Birthday!" There were at least 30 friends and acquaintances of mine pouring into the hallway, appearing from the kitchen and rising up from behind the chairs in the living room. I burst into tears of joy.

The party was a huge success. I received a number of presents which I could use in a practical way but, more than that, I felt deeply loved by my friends. Isabelle was the official photographer for the event and took many pictures of my smiling face as I opened the cards that were attached to the presents and read the loving words to the company gathered. It was a hallmark (no pun) day in my life. Carolyn gave me the gift of a glider ride in February at a local airport. Actually it was a ride for two, and she said in the card that it was for me and my brother. After the past four months of nausea and general malaise, I was delighted by this gift of adventure.

The day of the glider ride was bright and sunny. Ernie, Fay, Ken, Carolyn and I drove up to the tiny grass field called The Waterbury Airport in Thomaston, Connecticut. The sailplanes (as gliders are called by aficionados of the sport) were sitting, tilted over onto one wing at the end of the field. The wing-span was quite large. I felt a small knot in my stomach as I thought of the height involved in this adventure. I was surprised when I felt a warm sense of safety and relaxation come over me. I was changing...I had always been deathly afraid of height before. This was a new reaction to my old phobia.

Ernie and I—both over six feet tall—got into the rear section of the sailplane behind the pilot. He explained to us that the cable which was being walked back from the Cesna prop plane ahead of us would be attached to the nose of the glider and that at a certain altitude, we would hear a loud snap as he released the umbilical. We would then be "flying" on our own and, since a glider had no engine, we would not hear any other sounds. My knot momentarily reappeared and then I felt the strange and new sensation of acceptance that I had described earlier.

The Cesna sped up its engine and began moving down the field. There was a jolting tug as the cable came taut and our sailplane began to roll forward like a baby duck after its mother. The ground was bumpy and Ernie and I joked about hitting our heads on the roof of the cockpit but, without warning, all became smooth as the glider effortlessly rose above the airfield and we soared aloft. The tow plane took up rapidly to 2000 feet and we heard the prewarned snap as the cable was released by our pilot. We continued to soar upward on the warm drafts of rising air, heated by the afternoon sun, but the plane was almost completely silent. The only sound was an occasional creak in the structure and the rush of wind over the aerodynamic body of the plane. I felt like an eagle. My heart rose in my chest and I was joyously happy for the 45 minutes of the ride.

At one point before returning to the airstrip, the pilot turned slightly on his seat and said over his shoulder, "You're my last flight of the day. Would you guys like to do some loops?"

Ernie and I looked at one another and without any discussion, replied simultaneously, "No, thank you." We had experienced quite enough in the way of thrills for one day.

CHAPTER 14

In January of 1987 the days were especially cold for a man with short hair. I wore a hat all of the time and I still felt weak. I often recalled the despair I felt at the loss of my leg and from the cancer. Apparently tragedies tend to link themselves together in the human mind. Osteomyelitis resulting from the infections in my legs had persisted and was still a constant threat to my life. The thought that cancer could also recur was sometimes frightening to me. The resulting tissue damage from the chemotherapy—pulmonary fibrosis, Reynaud's disease, general weakness, constant tinnitus—were all continuing reminders of the fear and pain I had suffered. I had hated my long stays in the hospital and I had been thoroughly terrified by the hospital experiences. When I was in the hospital, I often found some kind of negative meaning for why I had to suffer. After returning from the final treatment to my home—surrounded by trees foretelling the end of summer—I tried to find some positive meaning for the same suffering. By January I was morose and confused. I was not having an easy time figuring out what changes, let alone higher purposes might have come from all that I had been through. As I pulled my scarf up on my winter coat in the 35 degree weather, I wondered if I had been given anything other than misery. A glint of hope rose in my chest as I thought of a positive outcome. The hope fell just as quickly. All I knew was that I did not want to die.

Laura Perls, my former supervisor and the co-inventor of Gestalt therapy, had told me after the accident that I would use my experience to help others who were handicapped and in wheelchairs. I had, indeed, done this. Colleagues and friends sometimes said supportive things like, "I'll bet your work as a therapist has really improved from all that you've been through." At first I would nod and think that they were probably correct. After all, some clients seemed to think that I was "more effective" because of my illness. I didn't know if that was merely the result of the difficulty they had projecting perfection upon me when I looked so sick or if I had actually changed in some way. Clients also said that I was "more approachable." This could have also been the result of their seeing my mortality. I had no certain evidence that, in fact, my personality or attitudes toward my work had changed. I thought, "I still do Gestalt therapy and I still do it in roughly the same way that I did it many years ago." Except for the fact that I was now able to run groups for the handicapped without seeming to be an "outsider," I was not finding my amputation or my cancer experience to be particularly enlightening or instructive.

As a child I had thought that suffering was some kind of punishment for a life badly lived. As an adult I imagined that suffering, once completed, would offer tremendous new insights into life and into the way in which one lived it, yet I was certain that I had not benefitted as a result of my pain. This was very discouraging and very uninspirational. I guess that I needed to deny that I had changed as a result of suffering. I think that some of my resistance was a natural part of my healing process. The first stage of grief is denial. I had felt denial in the hospital during my illnesses and injuries. My continuing need to deny significant change was a way of preventing me from moving forward through the rest of the grief process. By not acknowledging how I had changed, I was avoiding and denying my handicappedness and my mortality.

As the winter snows came and my strength returned, I began to alter my thinking. With the growth of my hair and the increase in body weight I felt a new enthusiasm about living. I looked ahead toward the life I had with a tremendous amount of gratitude and hope. I believed that I was given the chance to live once again in order to make the most of the life I had. I intended to do as much as I could with the time I had.

Toward the end of January I received a notice from the 52 Association for handicapped skiers announcing their ski week at Greek Peak at the end of February, and I immediately signed up for it. I also called a local travel agency and booked two tickets for Austria in April in order to take Carolyn on her "dream vacation" to ski in the Alps once again before she became too arthritic to attempt it. I was very proud that I had saved this money by working so hard throughout chemotherapy. I began to study very hard for the State Licensing Exam for Psychologists and took my books with me every morning to the diner where I went for breakfast.

Slowly but surely, I was making a comeback.

The drive to Greek Peak along route 84 and 17A was not very scenic and, anyway, my mind was on other things. I felt both a kind of enthusiasm about being with my friends skiing and some trepidation that I was too weak to be able to do much activity. I had gone to a local mountain on Friday just to try out a few runs and had fallen several times. My confidence was shaken a bit. I predicted that I might spend more time in the lodge than on the slopes but I was determined to have as much fun as I could under the circumstances.

I was greeted at the lodge by Mike, Sue, and Allen, all of them amputees. We embraced and they remarked on how short my hair was. I told them about my cancer experience and they were amazed that I was feeling well enough to come for a whole week of skiing. I told them that I would "ease into it" and went to the office to get the key to my chalet.

The apartment in which I stayed was shared by two other handicapped skiers. One of them, Wally, had lost his arm during the Korean War. He was bright and high spirited and immediately made me feel at home in our new surroundings. The chalet was beautifully furnished and even had a fireplace. We spent many nights after skiing, dozing on the couch in front of a comforting fire.

After unpacking my things and arranging my toiletries in the bathroom, I went down to the base lodge to sign up for ski lessons. I decided that the best way to get back into shape was to take some lessons from an instructor who would be willing to move at my pace. I asked for "private instruction." I was given a normal skier, Bill, who had been a soldier with the American Army ski troops stationed in Garmish in the Austrian Alps back in the 70s.

On Monday morning the frost nipped at my nose hairs as I stood, shivering, in the staging area waiting for my instructor. Bill shuffled over to me and introduced himself. He was darkly tanned from so much exposure to the sun and his face wrinkled, especially around his eyes, as he smiled. He was very patient with me and willing to take it quite slowly on the beginner and intermediate slopes as I relearned to carve turns and to exercise the unused muscles in my legs. After the first day I was thoroughly exhausted and immediately fell asleep after dinner in front of the fire in our chalet. As the week progressed, however, I seemed to recoup my strength quite rapidly, and by Wednesday evening, I was skiing as well as I had ever skied. Under Bill's tutelage, in fact, I was skiing considerably better.

At Greek Peak I spent the lunch breaks enjoying the company of my other amputee friends. We talked and told jokes and generally felt good humor about our various shortcomings. It was renewing to see them again. After lunch, when I had another hour before my next lesson, I took a run or two with my friends. It was very satisfying to show them how I was improving. They were very supportive of me and encouraged me to learn some tricks for racing. On Thursday, I decided to ask Bill to help me cut some time off of my slalom skiing. He brought me over to an advanced slope which had a complete slalom course on it. We concentrated on my carving closer and closer turns throughout the day's lessons. By the late afternoon I was able to lean quite strongly into the poles without fear of catching a ski tip and I was completely independent of my outriggers. I was now using regular ski poles for every run. Friday would tell how well I had learned my lessons.

At the end of the week I had a choice to ski in a race for handicapped persons or in another one for normal skiers. I opted for the latter. The race was called the Nastar. It is well known to skiers throughout the U.S.

As I entered the starting gate for my first run I was nervous. The exercise of the week was catching up with me, and every muscle in my body was aching. The official in the starting shed asked me if I was ready. "Yes," I said. "I'm not sure," I thought.

I pushed back against a block behind my poles lifting my skis in the air. The momentum carried me through the trip wire that started the timer and my skies plopped down on the crisp but rutted snow. I heard Bill's voice in the back of my mind yelling out to me to ski aggressively into the flag poles. I cut each one of them as closely as I could and hit every one of them with my arm as I shoved it out of the way. My skis moved smoothly over the snow and I felt my courage increase as I raced past the half-way marker. The air stung my face, but my glasses kept my eyes from watering. I was going faster than I had ever skied before as I crossed the finish line. I was so elated that I completely forgot to stop and look back to see my time. I just wanted to get to the lift line for my second and last run.

The second time was not very good, and I decided that I had released about all of the adrenalin I had available on the first run. I went back to the lodge and swapped stories about the week, the snow conditions and the races we had participated in that day. The food and hot coffee tasted great, and I no longer had any nausea eating the spiciest of dishes. When winners for the handicapped and Nastar races were announced I was told that I had won a Gold medal. I was breathless with excitement. Winning the Gold Medal in Nastar competition in a normal slalom race at Greek Peak topped off the growing feelings of well-being I started having before my trip.

As I packed my gear in my car that day and said goodbye to my friends, I felt like life was good and full of possibilities. During my drive home I had the knowledge that whatever life handed me I would somehow overcome it. This sense of survival-with-style was strong in me and is the hallmark of my way of dealing with tragedy even to this day.

I drove back from the skiing week. Spring was in the air. I felt wonderful. Now that I had proved to myself that I was improving physically, I would try to find a location for obtaining a year's post-doctoral residency. Things were looking up and there would be no stopping my ability to enjoy the life that had been given to me a second time.

Monday morning, I began my day by changing the dressing on my right foot (the skiing had removed some of the skin from my heel), soaking my artificial leg socket with alcohol to prevent infections, changing my stump stockings, putting on the leg to go to the bathroom to take a quick bath, coming back to the bedroom to get my clothes, taking off my leg to get dressed and finally putting the leg back on to go out to the kitchen to make breakfast. The morning procedure took over an hour.

By 10:00 I was ready to see clients. I only had two scheduled that day. My practice had naturally declined to just 16 people and I could afford to take huge chunks of time off to study or do other things around the house. I walked upstairs to greet my first client.

The spring sun sat warmly upon my shoulders as I stood in the front yard. I had spent a great deal of the recovery time after being in the hospital in the house and in my office. Unlike the office I had used in Ridgefield which had large windows looking out on the forest behind the cottage on Rainbow lake, this larger room was in my basement. It took our first summer in the new house for me to build the professional space. I had designed it just the way I wanted it, furnished it comfortably and gave it warm, even lighting. Even though I had built artificial windows in the dry walls of the office and some clients thought that we were on the first floor, I *knew* better.

I took a deep breath and inhaled the warm air. I could begin to smell the earth drying in the sun. The promise of white and purple crocuses could be seen in the succulent, green stalks that were pushing their way through the broken soil. The daffodils, too, were beginning their journey upward toward the sunlight, though with much smaller buds of pale green. I knew the scientific word, "phototropism," the tendency for plants to seek the source from which they would get the energy to manufacture chlorophyll—their own food. Feeling less scientific, however, I merely thought, "Ah...rebirth" as the light blue Toyota pulled into the driveway.

My client sat nervously on the large black couch and fumbled with her handkerchief. She had been crying a great deal. Her eyes were puffy and swollen. She was having difficulty coordinating her ideas and often changed the subject as if her brain simply could not maintain its neural focus. I recognized the symptoms of Major Affective Disorder with the probability of a personality disorder, but I was never one to substitute a diagnosis for the necessity of staying in the present moment with the client and working on whatever came up.

Joanne was a 32-year-old middle executive at one of the major corporate headquarters located in the Danbury area. She was presently in the Master of Business Administration program at a local university. She always dressed very well—impeccably, in fact. That day in March was no exception. She sat back on the soft couch, carefully smoothing her silk, calf-length dress with the oriental print, crossed her legs, dangling one very expensive leather shoe on the edge of her toes and leaned to one side against the mink coat on her left. Her long, brown hair was perfectly coiffed and, except for her crying, her makeup was done with the care of a model. Occasionally, she dabbed at her tears with a laced hanky.

"Joanne, if your depression could talk to me right now, what would it tell me?"

"What?"

"If your sadness could speak for you, Joanne, what would it say?"

"Oh...I don't know. I suppose it would say, I'm tired of being depressed."

"Tired of being depressed? Have you always been depressed?"

"Yeah...no, not really...I mean, I have been depressed for what seems like a very long time. I don't understand why....But, every day I feel like I'm no good or something like that." She squirmed in her seat as if she could not seem to get comfortable.

"Un huh. Depression can make you feel like you are worth less than you are. That's one of the symptoms of depression. Have you felt better about yourself when you were not depressed?" I leaned back into my hard metal chair and tilted the chair onto the two rear legs.

"No...that's the point. I have always felt like I was never good enough but I only started feeling really lousy in the past year."

"What happened a year ago?"

"Nothing terrible. In fact, it was something which I should feel really good about." Joanne flashed a momentary expression of fear during this statement.

"What's that?"

"I finished my bachelor's degree in business."

"Yeah...go on."

"Well, I was really happy for a while after I got my degree but now...now I feel real shitty again."

"You feel like shit?"

"Yep."

"Do you feel shitty or like you *are* shit?"

(Smiling to herself, she crossed and recrossed her legs) "...like I *am* shit. That's it. I feel worthless." Her eyebrows furrowed and her face wrinkled up for a new bout of tears. She dabbed daintily at the salty escapees and frowned when she noticed the black smudge of mascara on the edge of her hanky. She rubbed at the lace with a facial tissue which she had taken from the box I always leave on or near the couch.

"...and you felt worthless *before* you had your depression?"

"Of course. I have always felt worthless."

Having an insight, I replied, "Who are you trying to impress?"

"Huh? What's that?"

"I said, 'Who are you trying to impress?'"

"Nobody..." (a pause of 15 seconds occurred here. Joanne leaned forward onto her knees, both feet on the floor and looked pensive) "...well...I have always wanted to impress my dad."

"Joanne, would you be willing to try something that might help you to deal with some of your depressed feelings?"

"Huh?...Yeah, sure. What's that?"

"We can sometimes deal with someone who is not here in the office by imagining that this person *is* here. I will put another chair opposite to you and I would like you to imagine that your father is there in that chair. O.K.?" (As I said this I stood and walked over to one of my free chairs and arranged it in front of Joanne.)

"O.K....but I still don't get it."

"You don't have to do anything perfectly, Joanne." (I saw her face brighten at this instruction). "I would just like to see how you would interact with your father if he were here in this chair."

"All right....I'll try it." She straightened on the couch and adjusted her skirt so that there were no wrinkles in it.

I had an idea. I began with an instruction to her. "I'd like you to begin by saying, 'Dad...how do I look now?'"

Joanne looked at me with her bloodshot eyes. They widened slightly and she bit down on her bottom lip.

"What's happening?"

"I should say that?" She emphasized the word "that."

"You don't have to say anything in particular, Joanne. That is just a suggestion of mine. Would you be willing to try it?"

She stared ahead at the empty chair and her gaze became transfixed on the imagined figure of a man who must have been quite tall. "Dad. Do I look O.K. now?" Immediately Joanne put her hands to her face and began sobbing.

"What happened when you said that, Joanne?"

She could not answer me at first. Her sobbing became much louder and she kept trying to clean her face of the 'unsightly' tears. Her fingers instinctively rubbed the mascara from beneath her eyes and when she regained some of her composure, she straightened her hair. "I didn't say it the way you suggested...."

"That's O.K."

"...but I did feel something at that moment. It was like he was looking at me like I was ugly or something."

"Like you were ugly or like you didn't measure up?"

"Yeah...that's more like it...like I didn't measure up to *his* standards. He always found fault with me. He still does." Joanne's voice became harsh and caustic.

"What did he think of your Bachelor's degree?"

"Well that's just it. He never came to the graduation and he never sent me any card of congratulations or anything. When I called him a week later, he grunted something about my brother...you know, the one with the doctor's degree, and he said I'd have to get back to school for my Master's."

"You are in school for your Master's degree." She nodded. "Do you want to be there?"

Tears ran uncontrolled down her face. This time she did not try to block them from coming or even wipe them away. Her nose was running when she said to me, "No I don't. I think I have to do it to get him [jerking her head in the direction of the empty chair] to appreciate me."

"Tell him [nodding in the same direction] what you think of this situation."

Turning angrily toward the chair she spat out, "I hate it! You bastard." She paused as if waiting for a lightning bolt to descend from the ceiling. Seeing none, she continued. "You never thought I was as good as Daniel. I have always worked so hard to get your attention but it never does any good. What do I have to do to get you to like me?"

"Change chairs, Joanne, and show me what your father would say back."

She moved with some hesitation to the empty chrome-and-vinyl chair. As she sat down, her body seemed to rise to new heights. Her face looked imperious, haughty. "You stupid girl. You'll never be like Danny. *He's* really something. *He* became a physician...a surgeon. While you...you pathetic creature...you are merely a low-level supervisor in a chemical company. I told you that you'd never amount to anything." 'He' leaned forward on these last words and shook his finger at Joanne. Then he sat back, straightened his suit and seemed to reach for an imaginary breast pocket, take out a cigarette case, push the button, and extract one of its contents. The 'cigarette' was padded on the case and then brought to 'Dad's' mouth in a casual but calculated way, as if he were measuring each movement for effect.

"Dad, how do you feel right now as you look at Joanne's tears?"

"Ummmm...powerful. Yes. That's it. I feel powerful and...uh... *correct!*"

"...and that is something that is important for you to feel—important and correct."

"Yes it is. I need to feel correct...to feel...I don't know. I just know that I need to be correct."

"Change chairs and become Joanne again." She moved very slowly back to the couch and as she sat down, she seemed to crumple into a small heap. She reached over and pulled her fur coat across her belly and held it to her.

I inquired, "Did you hear what Dad said to you and how he felt about his impact on you?"

"Yes, I did. I feel crushed. He is sooo powerful! I have always felt inadequate in front of him...so...helpless."

"Would you be willing to try something further? Would you stand in front of the couch and face him in the chair from a standing position?"

"O.K." Joanne smoothed her dress again, fluffed her hair, wiped her face with her hanky and then stood before her 'father.'

I watched the way in which she postured herself. I could see that she was leaning back on her heels and would easily fall over onto the couch if pushed. I also noticed that there was a collapse in her chest created by her curving the spine outward like a case of lordosis.

"Joanne. Would you please become aware of your posture and please don't change it." She did as I instructed and seemed to visibly fight the urge to straighten up.

"I don't like the way I'm standing. My father would criticize it. He would say, 'Stand up straight, Joey.'"

This is the first time I had heard the name which Dad had called his daughter. I immediately felt like I was listening to the father talking to a son.

"Joey...tell your father how hard it has been for you to live up to his expectations of you."

She spent the next three or four minutes giving a diatribe of incidents in which he had found her lacking. The more she went on, the more I was certain that I was listening to a young boy responding to his father. I interrupted, "Joanne, tell your dad how hard it is for you to be another son to him."

She buckled at the knees as if hit in the chest. She fell backward and landed on her mink. She immediately turned to the side and burst into another round of tears. I watched her with great compassion and knew that she had been deeply self-injured as a child. She had been expected to be a boy for her father and to become the second in a series of male successes by becoming as accomplished as the first-born boy, Daniel. Not only could she never live up to the incredible needs of the father for perfection and achievement, but she would, whatever she accomplished, never achieve becoming a boy, no matter how she pulled in her chest. I waited for some of the crying to subside.

"That last idea seemed to hit you hard. Did that mean something to you?"

"The first thing I remember my father buying for me when I was a child was a baseball glove," she said with irritation. "I was always dressed in girl's clothes and told to be neat and pretty but the toys he kept buying me were always boys' things...like Tonka trucks and guns and stuff like that. My aunt Angelina was the only person who saw my needs as a child. If it wasn't for her I wouldn't have gotten a doll for Christmas."

"So here is one of the binds that your father put you in: 'Look like an attractive, perfectly made-up woman but achieve like Daniel'...in effect, 'don't be yourself whatever that may turn out to be.' Is that right?"

She nodded and began to cry again.

I interrupted, "Joanne, would you tell your father what you think of these messages?"

She immediately stood back up in front of 'his' chair, left her silk skirt wrinkled, placed her fists squarely upon her hips and spoke in a firm, low voice. "You have no right to control me like this. Who do you think you are...God? I already have a God and He is the only one for whom I have to live a good life. I don't want to live my life for you any longer. It is too difficult...no...*impossible!* I'm tired of 'dancing as fast as I can' for you [a quote from a famous book about a driven, self-disordered woman]. I don't know how yet but I'm going to start living my life for myself now. I want to be somewhat successful in my job, but I don't want that damn Master's degree and I'm perfectly content where I am in my job. I have plenty of opportunity for advancement in my company—Sally is V.P. in charge of marketing and she only has a Bachelor's degree. I can't..."

"...won't..."

"Right. I won't live up to your expectations of me. I am not the person that Daniel is and I DON'T WANT TO BE!"

As she spoke on this occasion her body was poised quite differently. She was standing with her weight placed half way between the front and back of her feet, her knees were slightly bent but her body was erect and flexible, her chest was not thrust forward but it was normally positioned and her back was without curvature. She appeared uncollapsed, flexible, yet strong.

"Joanne, would you again bring your awareness to your posture without changing it?"

She dropped her head slightly to look down at the way she was standing. She took survey of the position, smiled broadly, looked over at me and winked.

"You like the way you look?"

"I sure do. I feel strong…stronger than I have ever felt in my life."

"Are you also aware that your dress is wrinkled, your makeup is smudged and your hair disheveled?"

Smiling broadly, "Yep…and I don't give a fuck!"

"Uuuuuh (I inhaled). Such language from a lady!" I joked.

She laughed from the belly, finished the session, and began what would become a year's work on regaining all of the missing pieces of herself which she had given away in the process of becoming 'Daddy's little boy.' Another client was ready to remedy her childhood injuries. I, too, was well on my way to being healed of my own wounds.

AFTERWORD

I have been a psychotherapist for others for 19 years and an EMT since 1982. In the early years of my work as a therapist, I often worried about my abilities as a clinician. I worked very hard to learn the art and science of healing others emotionally. When I first trained as an EMT, I again felt the desire to give to accident victims the best possible health care I could. For nearly a decade I have confronted the agony of being a patient and client as well as a provider of human services. From the hot dust, grease, and blood on a narrow Ridgefield road, through the fear and constant nausea in an oncology ward, to the cool, clear winter air rushing past my face on the side of a mountain, I have experienced the many varied twists and turns which life takes.

The survival of tragedy was, at first, a total loss of control: to God, to other healers, to the love and concern of my family and friends, to fate, to the strength of my internal, biological healing process. As I developed a conscious awareness of my precarious balance between life and death, survival became a need to resolve internal conflicts between parts of myself that wanted to place blame (on myself or others), deal with loss (or avoid dealing with it), and express anger (or retroflect the anger back upon myself and get depressed). It was also an emotional and physical fight against the injury or disease which ravaged my frame. In overcoming the lethargy of self-pity, the fear of childhood misbeliefs and the pain that racked my body on a daily basis, I survived a great internal struggle. By facing life as a gift to be persistently pursued, by opening up to the support of those who loved me and, most importantly for me, by returning with new conviction to my work as a helper and healer of others, I survived the external demands and terrors which tragedy brought. My work gave me the sense of purpose I needed to go on. It was, as well, a vehicle by which I could give others the precious gifts that had been given to me. Through my own wounding, suffering, and healing myself, and also by passing that persistent struggle for survival onto clients and accident victims, I have faced life literally from both sides. Helping others, however, was and still is one of the strongest supports that I use to survive and to grow as a healer.

9 780893 919733

Printed by Libri Plureos GmbH in Hamburg,
Germany